HEALING
TIMES

A PERSONAL WORKBOOK

LOUISE GIROUX

HEALING

TIMES

A PERSONAL WORKBOOK

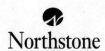

Northstone

Editor: Michael Schwartzentruber, Dianne Greenslade
Cover design: Lois Huey-Heck
Consulting art director: Robert MacDonald

Permissions:
Cover tapestry: Bolcena #033, used with permission of Avant Garde Fabrics, Canada.

Northstone Publishing Inc. is an employee-owned company, committed to caring for the environment and all creation. Northstone recycles, reuses and composts, and encourages readers to do the same. Resources are printed on recycled paper and more environmentally friendly groundwood papers (newsprint), whenever possible. The trees used are replaced through donations to the Scoutrees For Canada Program. Ten percent of all profit is donated to charitable organizations.

Canadian Cataloguing in Publication Data
Giroux, Louise, 1951-
    Healing Times

    Includes bibliographical references.
    ISBN 1-55145-089-5

    1. Self-actualization (Psychology). I. Title.
BF637.S4G57   1997   158'.1   C96-910726-9

Published by Northstone Publishing Inc.

Printing
9 8 7 6 5 4 3 2 1

Printed in Canada by
Friesen Printers
Altona, MB

Northstone

DEDICATION

*It is with admiration and respect that I
dedicate this "work" book to all the men
and women who summon the courage to
undertake their own healing.*

TABLE OF

CONTENTS

CHAPTER 4
INNER CHILD

CHAPTER 5
SEXUALITY

CHAPTER 6
COUPLE RELATIONSHIPS

CHAPTER 7
CAREER

CHAPTER 8
PARENTING

CHAPTER 9
TOPSY-TURVY: ILLNESS

CHAPTER 10
ME & YOU, YOU & ME

CHAPTER 11
DIVORCE/BLENDED FAMILIES

CHAPTER 12
RECYCLING THE CIRCLE

CONCLUSION

FOREWORD

Healing Times: A personal workbook is, as the subtitle suggests, a hands-on resource aimed at the individual who wants to increase his or her self-awareness and day-to-day functioning. It is also a resource for the professional who wants a structural guide to assist him or her in addressing, with clients, emerging themes from the past that can be recycled in new and helpful ways for the client.

Healing Times contains much that will prove helpful to the reader: the practical "to do" exercises, the case examples, and the reflective nature of the text itself. Even more than these, I know the workbook to be born out of the lived encounters of Louise with her own clients and her own personal work. This material has been lived through and found to have worked in the everyday experiences of its author and ordinary people.

Healing Times provides ways for persons to address the recurring themes of their past, and to recycle these themes in ways that can lead to changed perspectives, behavior and patterns, and feelings. *Healing Times* is developmental in that it starts with early childhood experiences and brings you to the present. The resource is cyclical in that it assists the user in the awareness that our endings represent new beginnings, places from which we venture with new awareness, skills, and confidence.

Healing Times is a resource you will find yourself reaching for again and again, each time to discover something rich and enriching.

Rev. Melvin Rose B.A. S.T.M.
Clinical Director and Teaching Supervisor (C.A.P.P.E.)
The Pastoral Institute of Northern Ontario

PREFACE

While I underwent my own therapeutical process, I discovered that "doing the work" was the only effective way to get on with my life. What I also discovered was a serious lack of tools, exercises, and the like, with which I could process "the work."

Years later, when I interned in psychotherapy, a similar awareness was raised. Those people doing the work were the ones who healed quickly and effectively. However, there was a lack of practical and simple tools and exercises available to the world of therapy. I began to make use of my teaching and creative skills to think up exercises.

Thus, this workbook was born. It could just as easily have been called "Doing the Work." Its content is the fruit of personal work done, as well as my clients' work.

Unfortunately our technological society does not prepare us well for work that requires time, patience and persistence. You may savor a meal, cooked in three minutes in your microwave, but let me assure you there is no quick way to do the work that is involved in recycling, or redefining, one's self. This process of recycling, of recovering and healing from problematic situations or incidents is available to every one of us. The question is not, "Will it work?" but rather, "Am I committed to giving the time and emotional energy necessary?"

My hope is that you will find this workbook enjoyable rather than painful. I have attempted to create exercises that are play and enjoyment oriented, since I am an advocate of lightening-up our lives.

I wish you much success in your journey of healing.

Shalom
Louise Giroux

NOTE TO
READERS

All of the cases reported in this workbook are an accurate reflection of what actually took place in people's lives. However, in every case, identifying characteristics have been changed to protect confidentiality. Occasionally the cases of two or more people have been amalgamated into one, for a more effective presentation.

The author welcomes letters from readers.
Write to: Louise Giroux
Box 172, Station Q
Toronto, ON
M4T 2M1

CHAPTER 1

DOING THE

WORK

"It's hard work but somebody has to do it...and it must be me."
– Louise Giroux

So often I have heard my clients say, "Tell me what to do... I want to do the work...I want healing." My reply is, "You're doing it."

The *you* in you're doing it

This is the important dimension of ownership. All of us work through our own situations and even if we are fortunate enough to have the most competent of professionals to guide us, we, personally, must take ownership of our problems, our process and our healing. The work has to be ours.

The *doing* in you're doing it

Doing the work is not limited to physical activity. Its scope encompasses your thoughts, your feelings, as well as your actions. When you read, when you write, when you verbalize, when you think, when you visit, you are doing the work. It has indeed a nebulous character at times, while in other instances it communicates a real sense of something being done.

The *it* in you're doing it

It refers to the work which in effect might take on a variety of characteristics. What the work involves is the action, the thought or the feeling processed in order for resolution or healing to take place. You will experience some sort of change when the work is successfully completed. You will know that your endeavors have been successful when the hurt or the discomfort goes away. Remember, there is no specific time frame, no deadline and no magic map. Instead, you can be ready for a courageous, concerted effort toward your healing process.

TYPES OF ISSUES

These are a few typical issues or situations that could warrant "doing the work."
• grieving the loss of a person who dies
• grieving the loss of a relationship
• chronic illness, whether an emotional, mental, or physical challenge
• family of origin conflict
• low self-esteem
• career and productivity

- parenting and/or or stepparenting children
- interpersonal relationships
- sexuality
- marital conflict
- inner child unresolved issues
- sexual activity and preference

SIGNS OR SYMPTOMS

These are some of the signs or symptoms that would indicate that something is not quite right with you. They may be comments made by others or they may be in the form of your thoughts or simply your own observations.

- Since she died, I walk around with such a hole in my heart.
- Even if I chose to leave my marriage, all I do now is cry.
- At first, my new wife and I were honeymooners; now all we do is argue over the kids.
- Who pulled the plug on my health? I want to kill somebody.
- Whenever there's a family get-together, I get apprehensive.
- I need a change in my job; I am too old to start somewhere else.
- My son is getting into trouble at school. I must be a bad mom.
- I swear my mother is harder to handle than my kids were.
- My friendships are superficial and don't last long.
- My husband and I both think about separating. Would we be better off?
- Out of nowhere, the other night as I watched a movie, in my mind's eye I remembered Mr. Smith fondling me when I was about eight years old. I freaked out in the middle of the movie.
- Whenever I open up to my partner, I feel I'm not being heard.
- I am totally fed up with always doing for others. When is it going to be my turn?
- Each year around Christmas time, I get really depressed.
- I envy the women who claim their homosexuality and I tend to think that I am leaning toward that myself. It would kill my family.
- Our sex life sounds like a broken record. I sing the blues because I never feel like it and my husband sings "I can't get no satisfaction."
- No matter what I achieve, there is always an undercurrent of "I'm not as good as others."

CASE STUDY

Joe is an angry man; he is obnoxious and sarcastic with the therapist. When she asks why he is here, since he certainly does not act like someone who wants to be in therapy, his voice softens.

Joe does not have much confidence in therapy; if it weren't for his wife giving him an ultimatum, he would not be here. Lately, the bottle has been his refuge. Although he drinks daily and progressively more and more, he rejects other people's opinion that he has a problem. The therapist responds that maybe the alcohol is not the problem, that living is the problem. Obviously, Joe has been programed with all of the negative connotations of "drunk" and "bad" and "be a man and quit." When the therapist begins to explain how alcoholism operates, what it is, what it is not, Joe is amazed at his own discoveries. This is a license for Joe to explore his situation with less fear than before.

As part of the exploration and treatment, the therapist questions Joe about anything and everything. A rapport builds between the client and the therapist and, what at the beginning seemed like an odd combination, slowly develops into an intimate professional rapport. The therapist often outlines the boundaries that each of them needs to maintain so as not to allow the therapy to be destructive.

Obviously, there is a lot of unfinished business in Joe's past: ungrieved deaths and other losses, a childhood on the welfare system, a learning disability. The therapist will treat him with inner child work once Joe is strong enough to process it.

As the months pass, Joe's typical comment, "Well here I go into the torture chamber," takes on more and more meaning. Indeed he does work which is painful, work that changes his life and the lives of those he loves and knows.

A few times, when the therapist had assigned "homework" to be completed, Joe came back with excuses. His therapist confronted him on this, forcing him to either commit or not to "doing the work." Whenever he played mind games with her, the therapist was quick to challenge Joe, who grew to respect his therapist.

At one point, Joe decided that he was cured and wanted to terminate the sessions. The therapist went along with him, knowing full well that the work was not completed. Sure enough, within a few weeks, Joe returned for another session. It was a learning experience, part of doing his work, of course. When Joe invited his family to join him in session, they refused to go; this was disappointing for him. The therapist assisted Joe as he claimed responsibility for his own work and detached himself from other people's opinions.

Of course, the cycle of therapy hit Joe like a ton of bricks. He experienced exhaustion, sadness, anger, euphoria, extreme highs and lows, and other symptoms that led him to believe that he was getting worse instead of better. The therapist's image was that of a surgical procedure: "It's right after the surgery and the removal of the gall bladder that you feel as though you were better off before; wait it out..." Above all, Joe had developed a trust in his therapist that allowed him to keep moving on.

At one session, Joe brought a flower for his therapist and they discussed the healthy boundaries that they had for each other. It remained clear that they had a professional relationship.

While shopping one day, the therapist bumped into Joe, who had by then stopped his therapy. At first the therapist waited for acknowledgment from her former client and, when it came, they chatted for a few minutes. Joe introduced her to his wife and, as he did, the therapist observed a gleam in his eyes, an aliveness, a message that said "Life is okay."

EXERCISE IN SONG

The song is *We'll Reach the Stars Tonight* by Rita MacNeil.

One of the most important motivators to doing the work is goal-setting. It gives you a sense of purpose and something to shoot for. You need to gather the tools necessary to reach your goal; they might be assets of your own personality, input from other people in your life, objects you have at your disposal, etc. It is also recommended that you draw a road map for yourself.

As well as being equipped with the proper tools, you will need to chart out a path for yourself to follow. This might entail which telephone call to make first or which person to see. Make sure your goals are realistic and your expectations appropriate.

After you have listened to the song selection, think about and chart a goal plan for yourself relating to the work you might want to accomplish for your situation.

Example

my goal: *Sarah*

issue: *ineffective communication with my teenaged daughter*

goal: *to diminish the constant verbal fights that occur between us*

tools: *my willingness to better the situation*
my daughter's knowledge that I really care about her
a book, Please Understand Me
an interest group on parenting
my daughter's study week coming up

road map: *read my resource book*
get support from others in the parenting group
give her more positive stroking
invite her to take a 2-day trip with me
engage in a meaningful conversation, express my concerns
and ask her for input

expected outcome: *improvement of the communication between my*
daughter and me

Remember: It is far better to have small goals that are achievable than to have large goals which can never be achieved. It is a priority to set a goal, any goal, that we can reach in a limited time. Once the sense of accomplishment of that goal sets in, our attitude about ourselves begins to blossom. Good luck.

my goal:

issue:

goal:

tools:

road map:

expected outcome:

EXERCISE IN FILM

The selection for this chapter is *Duet for One*, directed by Andrei Konchalovsky. In making the film selection, I sought out a success story. It would be naive to believe that all persons who do their work rise from the ashes and succeed as well as the heroine did. However, the film depicts a reality in terms of the process involved in therapy. Watch the film and then do the writing exercise that follows.

Exercise: Doing the work

1. How does the relationship between the heroine and her therapist develop?

2. What does her work consist of?

3. Which changes do we observe as she does her work?

Prescription: Journaling

Why journal

In the prologue to my autobiography, *Recycled: A Story of Hope*, I spoke about writing, not to be understood, but rather to understand. This is what journaling is all about; it is a tool with which we come to understand. Once we have an understanding of what happens to us, why it happens and how we experience what happens to us, we may begin to make changes. Awareness precedes change. The suggestions I recommend on the topic of journaling are but a very few of the unending possibilities.

Where to journal

Select a book or notepad that appeals to you, also a pen or pencil that suits you; your computer might be appropriate as a choice for you. I recommend that you choose a medium that validates who you truly are.

What to journal

Anything and everything. Whatever is on your mind, in your heart or needs sorting out. If you are seeing a professional, he or she may assign things to journal about.

When to journal

Some people keep journaling all day long. I recommend daily, at a regular time. By recording each day at a set time, the procedure becomes habitual and you will have a better chance of doing it routinely.

How to journal

Write primarily for yourself and be spontaneous. Forget about grammar and spelling and all those "perfect" habits. You can jot down ideas, write letters, compose poems or essays, whatever floats your boat.

Processing a journal

So what can we do with our journaling? Amazingly enough, the journaling in itself is sufficient in some cases. If you find a need to process the material, you can do so with a confidant or with a professional. You will be amazed at your recurring themes and images, at the words you use to describe your feelings and thoughts.

PRESCRIPTION: PARENTHESIS"ING"

Parenthesis"ing" is a crucial technique by which you can remain safe and go on with your life and day-to-day responsibilities while doing the work. If you have ever left a session with a professional or a session with a confidant, you are aware of what the aftermath may be like in terms of feelings and thoughts. The following exercise is designed to assist you in leaving the content of the session behind you for a while, while you resume your "normal" life.

Materials
pencil and paper
a few moments
a "tuck away" place

Immediately after finishing a session, take out your pencil and paper; jot down very briefly (one sentence or less) the main thrust of what it is you need to put away for now, in order to resume your normal activities. For example: my love/hate thing with Mom, or my sadness over John. Take the paper and fold it. On top of it, write a time and a place when you expect to be able to reopen this issue. Tuck the paper away where it will be safe, yet accessible – your wallet, pocket, etc. Go on with your normal routine; when it is appropriate, you will simply go back to your note and reopen the issue.

PRESCRIPTION: EENIE-MEENIE-MYNIE-MO/CHOOSING A THERAPIST

The Ten Commandments

1. Know what you need.
2. Shop around for a therapist.
3. Be verbal and assertive.
4. Fire the therapist if necessary.
5. Check out boundaries.
6. Watch for the therapist who does their own work during your sessions.
7. Validate the therapist.
8. Be aware that you will change.
9. Always pay your bill.
10. Notify the therapist if you need to cancel a session.

Hopefully you have joined those of us who have demystified professional health care workers. In our times, and not a moment too soon, we give ourselves permission to choose our services as well as freedom to negotiate and to change the services if they have become of no use. Your therapist is hired by you to provide a service. Work on developing an effective professional relationship with him or her; you will discover that most professionals desire the same thing. In every occupation, you will discover incompetency, lack of experience and knowledge, or just plain miserable people. Treat yourself to the best possible self-care help available to you...you're worth it.

PRESCRIPTION: SUPPORT SYSTEM

Doing the work is hard work. Persons doing their work are apt to feel quite alone and in need of emotional support. I encourage you to network with a selected few while you are working. If I recommend a "selected" few, it is because I want to discourage dependency building. Your support network can be absolutely anyone whose role it is to be present in your life. There is no need to set specific times for meeting and sharing with your support; simply contract once with them that #1) you are doing some work and #2) their support is important to you. A note dropped in the mail, or a quick phone call is often the perfect thing. While you do your work, you will avoid isolation by networking with others. Give yourself the gift of support from others.

PRESCRIPTION: CHAMPIONS

Materials
a clear idea of an issue that needs work
a list of three of your champions

When you are doing the work, you will need to be inspired by champions. We all have a few of them, whether they be political heroes, spiritual leaders, sports heroes, or family members – alive or deceased. Whether or not your champions have experience in your particular type of work is irrelevant. The idea is to tap into your champions' energy and minds to find clarity in your own dilemmas.

For example: "I wonder what piece of advice or consolation Patti Duke would have to offer me now that my depression has hit worse than ever..." (For information about Duke, consult *A Brilliant Madness*.)

You can enter into "mind dialog" with your champions as to how they would handle any particular aspect of the work situation. This exercise is remedial in cases where we feel isolated, confused or weak. Our champions can inspire us if we read their stories and their courage energizes us. I suggest you actually write to your champions if you can; you might be surprised at their responses.

My champions:

1.

2.

3.

Prescription: Come Here, Kid

In the fourth chapter of this workbook, I suggest some exercises that deal with "inner child work." However, it might be good to check out the nature of this type of work now, as well as process your need to do some work in this area.

Because inner child work is essential to all courses of therapy in my opinion, I recommend an attempt at it. It is because of the fact that "we are where we come from" – that our childhood has shaped us, no matter how far we think we have distanced ourselves from it – that getting in touch with our inner child is imperative. After all, whether you choose to welcome him or her, your inner child is always with you for the ride. Why not learn to accept this child and work with them instead of against them? Do the work in the inner child realm slowly, cautiously and preferably with someone to coach you.

Do not do inner child work if
- You are feeling low in emotional, mental or physical energy.
- You are using drugs or alcohol.
- It is a means of avoiding the here-and-now issues that need attention.
- You cannot find support.
- The therapist is not experienced with it.
- You think that your "adult" cannot handle it right now.

Exercise

The following series of questions will raise your awareness in the area of inner child work. It is a writing exercise which I suggest taking special quiet time to do. Journal what it is like for you to answer these questions – what do you feel, what do you think, what do you want – in general, what happens to you as you answer the questions.

1. (a) What major changes have happened in your family of origin in the last 20 years? For example, what births, deaths, marriages, departures or other changes in status occurred?

(b) How did family members react to these changes?

(c) How have you or your brothers and sisters been involved in these changes?

2. (a) What were some of the openly acknowledged and spoken rules in your family?

(b) What were some of the unspoken rules about having and expressing feelings?

3. (a) What role did you play?

(b) Identify the role of other siblings.

4. (a) What tendencies towards illness did you become aware of?
For example, alcoholism, depression, etc.

5. What are the rules in your partner's family of origin and how do they conflict with your own?

6. (a) What happened to the level of anxiety in your family when rules were broken? Who would begin to object, make an issue of the behavior, or become anxious? For example, if anger was not acceptable, what would happen if someone began to openly express anger in the family? How would it be controlled?

(b) What rules do you think you are still observing? How do you react when they are broken?

Prescription: I'm My #1 Fan

Don't panic. This is not an exercise in narcissism...*au contraire*. It is an exercise in validation and building of self-esteem. The undercurrent of many difficulties we encounter is due, to some extent, to some form of low or wounded self-esteem. As part of creating the climate for doing the work, as well as for maintaining our focus while we do the work, self-validation is crucial.

Exercise

Write a love letter to yourself; make it a tribute to your courage and willingness to work at your own healing.

Dear Me,

Love, Self

"Before you begin, understand that healing is neither immediate nor linear. You don't start at point A (pain) and rush to point B (recovery) in a straight line. You need time to travel up one day, down a little the next, and perhaps up again the third. Healing occurs as you walk the hills and meadows. Be patient and gentle with yourself on your journey."

– P. McConnell, A Workbook for Healing

RECOMMENDED RESOURCES

1. Bentley, Timothy. *The 90 Second Therapist*. Summerhill Press, Toronto, 1988
2. Chapman, Joyce. *Journaling for Joy*. Newcastle Publishing Co., Inc. 1991
3. Cooper, Robert. *Stressmap*. Newmarket Press, New York, 1984
4. Daldrup, Beuttler, Engle and Greenberg. *Focused Expressive Psychotherapy*
   The Guilford Press, New York, 1988
5. Donovan, Dennis. *Addictive Behaviors*. The Guilford Press, New York, 1988
6. Giroux, Louise. *Recycled: A Story of Hope*
   Fenix Ryzing Associates, Sudbury, Ontario, 1995
7. Hanson, Peter, *The Joy of Stress*
   Hanson Stress Management Organization, 1985
8. ———. *Stress for Success*. Collins Toronto, 1989
9. Hodgson, Ray and Peter Miller. *Self-Watching*
   Methuen Publishings, Toronto, 1982
10. James and Jongeward. *Born to Win*
    Addison-Wesley Publishing Company, Don Mills, Ontario, 1976
11. Johnson, Catherine. *When to Say Goodbye to your Therapist*
    Simon and Schuster, New York, 1988
12. Johnson, Rheta Grimsley. *Good Grief*. Ravette Books, London, 1989
13. Kiley, Dan. *What to Do when He Won't Change*
    G.P. Putnam's Sons, New York, 1987
14. Lüscher, Max. *The Lüscher Color Test*
    Random House, New York, 1969
15. McKay M., M. Davis, and P. Fanning. *Messages*
    New Harbinger Publications, 1983
16. Miller, S., D. Wackman, E. Nunally, and P. Miller. *Connecting*
    Interpersonal Communication Programs, Inc. 1988
17. Palmer, Helen. *The Enneagram*
    Harper and Row Publishers, San Francisco, 1975
18. Powell, John. *Will the Real Me Please Stand Up?*
    Tabor Publishing, Valencia, CA, 1985
19. Sheehy, Gail. *Pathfinders*. Bantam Books, Toronto, 1981
20. Stewart, John. *Emotional First-Aid Manual*
    The Canadian Mental Health Association British Columbia Division, 1988
21. Tauber, Ezriel. *Self-Esteem*. Shalheves, New York, 1992
22. Wynn, J. C. *The Family Therapist*
    Fleming H. Revell Company, New Jersey, 1981

CHAPTER 2

FAMILY OF

ORIGIN

"The more intensively the family has stamped its character
upon the child, the more [the child] will tend to feel
and see its earlier miniature world again
in the bigger world of adult life."
– C.J. Jung

This chapter and the following chapter present the theme of family roles and family of origin. What was the general atmosphere in your family-of-origin system as you grew up? Each member within this system, whether related by blood or marriage, influences the interaction between all other members.

How did your family system set up its positions? Who played the eldest child? Was there a middle scapegoat? How did the youngest child act out his or her role? What was your position in the family and how was that experience for you?

It will be enriching for you to define your family role and especially to observe how you have carried over this role to your present relationships. Some of us leave home at a young age; some of us leave very slowly and progressively; some of us have only just left home; while others are still at home, that is to say, still maintaining the same dynamic in our adult lives.

CASE STUDY

Sam is a middle-aged man, anxious and lacking self-confidence. He reports having little to do with his family of origin, which consists of an older brother and a younger sister. As we sketch out his family of origin, we find that Sam was in the middle of two children. His siblings managed to get most of the attention from the parents: the eldest son gained recognition because he was perfect in everything he did, and the youngest daughter gained recognition because she was ill. As for Sam, his world consisted of books and television, in which he found refuge and connection. His parents would always say how he was so quiet, and no trouble at all.

Of course, the truth was that Sam was a lost child. He never felt connected to his siblings or to his parents. In therapy, we discovered that Sam had become caught in the middle between his mother and his father whenever Mom wanted to teach Dad how to be quiet. She would want Dad to learn, from Sam, how to occupy his time by himself. As we went through various snapshots that Sam had been asked to bring in, almost every photograph revealed Sam as an unsmiling, almost invisible member of the family, usually on the offset or in a corner.

Some of the colors that Sam preferred to wear were the dark hues and these were also found in the drawings he drew as a child. Sam had been suicidal on occasion and mainly depressed all his life. He reported being extremely isolated and not connected to anyone.

In his adult life, Sam had gravitated toward strong characters, elders of families, or to the weak and feeble, like his younger sister. Once again, he would be caught in the middle, the lost role, and very soon that relationship would end. He repeated his family of origin structure in adult relationships.

The awareness and the willingness with which he approached his therapy work led to success. For Sam, it meant an opening up of certain old emotional wounds and some grieving of the nurturing parents that he never had. After some rather emotionally surgical exercises, we found a new pattern of relating for Sam. He discovered that his family role could be altered and eradicated at this point. At the age of 47, Sam finally left home.

EXERCISE IN SONG

The chosen selection is *Places that Belong to You*, from the motion picture *The Prince of Tides*. Listen to the recording. It is a good place to begin the journey back. Try to be aware of your experience in your family of origin.

This is a letter writing exercise. Focus on yourself at age ten. Then, write a letter to each of your siblings, a letter in which you address your relationship with each one of them. If you were older than ten when younger siblings came along, write from that age. If you are an only child, address this issue in a letter to your parents. You could also write to a significant childhood friend, a surrogate sibling. The processing of these letters can be done with a confidant or a therapist or simply by yourself.

Everything about how you approach and actually perform this task, if you choose to do so, will reveal the way in which you experience your family of origin in your present life. Also, what you do with the writing, that is, whether you actually go over it with your family or not, will be of significance for you in your present life.

Dear _____,

Your sister (brother),

EXERCISE IN FILM

The film for this exercise is *The Prince of Tides*. As you view the movie selection, try to be aware of the pattern in this family of origin, the role of each of the three siblings as well as the parental dynamic in the family system. The emotional content of this film can be quite demanding, please take care of yourself by either watching with someone you can share with or with a professional.

This is a writing exercise. Answer each of the following questions as best you can. They will address the topics of sibling position and influence, of escape for emotional safety, as well as the effect of abuse on a family system. They will also address parent-child triangulation, that is, one parent uses the child to communicate with the other parent rather than communicating directly.

1. The mother says to different children, "You're my favorite, don't tell the others I told you this." How do you think this type of relationship affects the child to whom she is speaking ?

2. The father is a physical aggressor in the story line. How does mother deal with this man?

3. The eldest, responsible son becomes a criminal. How does he act out his family script?

4. How does Savannah escape the horror of her experience?

5. Savannah's protector is her twin. How does this role affect the leading character, the Prince of Tides?

6. What about the secrets in this family system? Are there any secrets in your family of origin?

7. How is it that the leading character recovers from his childhood through assisting in the therapeutical process for his sister?

VARIOUS EXERCISES

The following exercises will help you to focus on your family of origin pattern. If you have already done some of the suggested work, by now you probably have a better awareness of how it was, of how it possibly still is for you in this family. Whenever you discover pleasant memories, cherish them and focus on those also. These exercises are created to help in rediscovering old truths, discovering new truths and recording pleasant memories for yourself.

PRESCRIPTION: TRIANGLES

Triangulation is a pattern of relationship wherein three persons are interacting. These triangles may be of various angular degrees, thus creating different distances between members of the trio. Also, these triangles are not usually consciously constructed but rather a way in which persons relate within a system. As much as possible, we want to avoid triangulation, since it makes direct relating between two people almost impossible. In other words, someone communicates "around" or through another person, rather than to the person directly. Commonly, we observe triangles at some point between a child and his or her parents.

In the example below, Jessica is caught between her parents who each pull her their own way in their divorce, seeking loyalty from her. It is not healthy for any of them.

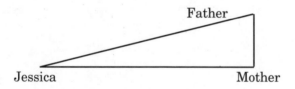

In the following example, Jessica is supported by one of her brothers and distanced from the other brother; she often has to babysit them, and so, the triangulation is frequent.

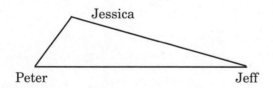

Exercise: My Triangles

Outline some of the triangles in your family of origin, as you perceive them. Notice the distances between yourself and the two other parties. Are you drawn into these triangles by someone else? Do you create them? How does this pattern of relationship exist in your adult relationships?

PRESCRIPTION: SNAPSHOT THERAPY

Photos reveal a wealth of information about you and about your family. One client recalled how she noticed that whenever there were family parties, the photographs revealed her acting as a mascot, always the clown. It was never so apparent to her as when she observed herself in the collection of photos. She had acted as the family clown for a very long time.

EXERCISE

Find a selection of family photos, preferably some in which you are at various ages. The ideal is a collection, where you can trace yourself from birth to the present. These are some of the questions you might ask yourself while you observe them or as someone looks at the photos with you.

- Whom are you with?
- What type of facial expression do you have?
- What about expressions of other members around you?
- What types of feelings get stirred for you as you look at any particular photo?
- Did you already have photos or did you search them out?
- Is there a period of your life where there aren't any photos?
- What sort of events were occurring around the taking of these photos? Observe people's posture.
- What things, objects or possessions appear with you in the photos?
- Is there an alignment of people in the photo? Any recurring order?
- Do you like yourself in the photos?
- How do the significant people in your life at present react to these photos?

PRESCRIPTION: SIBLING POSITION

Birth order has become a great way for us to discover some of our relational patterns. Depending on whether you are an older, a middle or a youngest child will affect how you relate to others. If you are from a family of more than three, you can very easily determine which position you held by taking a look at the script that accompanied your role. Your script is the "understood" way in which you were expected to behave; for example, the eldest child in a family is often expected to be "the responsible one." You may want to check out the recommended reading *Birth Order and You* which appears at the end of this chapter.

Not only do we grow with a defined role in sibling position, but we also may choose a partner who is either of a different, complementary position or same position. Often, the way in which we relate to this partner will be affected by the pattern we used with our sibling of the same sibling position as our partner. Of course, whether we are the youngest sister of older brothers, or the eldest sister of younger brothers, or a middle girl with an older brother and a younger brother, or any combination in terms of gender it will be interesting for us to trace. How did all of this affect us then? More importantly, how does this affect us now?

Materials
a willing adult with a sense of sibling position
a tape recorder and blank cassette
a few people who are willing to be interviewed

EXERCISE

Conduct a few interviews with various people that you know in order to ask them about their own sibling position and how that experience was for them. You can draw a chart also, to reveal which position order these people have chosen for their partner. It is a rich resource for experiencing belonging. Once you have discovered a few people who share your common sibling position, you may want to have a brainstorming session together, where you will share how the experience varied or was common for those members of the group. You could interview your partner to determine how they experience their position with you in your present relationship. If you are an only child, you may want to extend this to any significant relationships you had as a child and now have as an adult.

Prescription: Family Weather Map*

A) On the following page, draw a weather map of your family of origin in the space provided, using the symbol that best describes your family.

   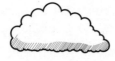   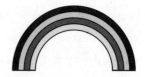

Sunshine represents a happy, healthy family.

Rainclouds represent extreme, unresolved conflict in a family system, what we term a dysfunctional family.

The rainbow represents that the family is experiencing difficulty, but active healing is happening – there is hope.

B) Above the picture of your family of origin, indicate an emotion that your family had difficulty in expressing, or in dealing with.

C) Below the picture, indicate a strength that your family has.

D) In the top left hand corner, indicate what the main role of the parents was.

E) In the top right hand corner, indicate who was a great influence in your life.

F) In the bottom left hand corner, describe the role of children in your family.

G) In bottom right hand corner write about a dream or a wish that you have for your family.

*This exercise is adapted from *In the Spirit of the Family,* The National Association of Treatment Directors, Calgary, 1989.

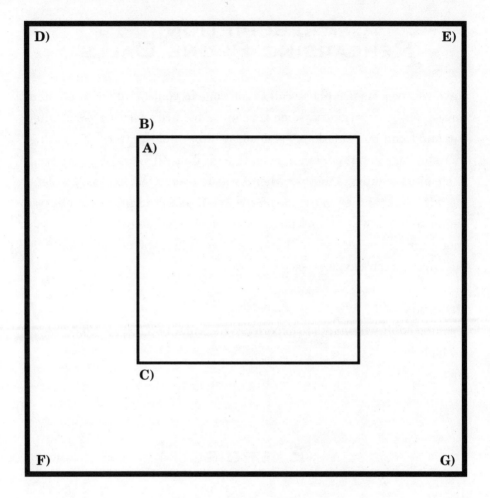

D)   E)

B)

A)

C)

F)   G)

What this type of weather picture can provide for you is a visual display of the atmosphere and the general feeling that prevailed in your family system. You might find it hopeful to think of a future state in which you would ideally want your family of origin to be. Some of us are fortunate enough to communicate effectively with our family of origin; it is precious for us to share with them the discoveries that we make. If the awareness that you raise translates into difficult emotion for you, seek the assistance of a professional in order to deal with your past and in order to live well within the family of origin to which you belong. Enjoy leaving home, enjoy learning to visit now and again, in a healthy manner.

PRESCRIPTION:
REHEARSING PHONE CALLS

Have you ever made a phone call to someone in your family of origin and, consequently, experienced some turmoil afterward? This happens when our mind and our emotions get hooked into an old pattern of relating; therefore, speaking to mother, even though I am 40 years old, may seem to me like speaking to mother when I was ten years old. One way of dealing with this, and of individuating yourself as an adult, is to rehearse phone calls. You will be conscious of your level of individuation by how you keep your cool or by how well you avoid getting involved emotionally in the other person's experience.

Materials
a willing adult who wants to experience individuation (separation)
a telephone
a pad and pencil

EXERCISE

Simply write down exactly what your message will be, taking into account the possible message you will receive. Whenever you feel yourself yielding to the responses and straying from your intended message, read back what you have written, that is, get into your message again, letting go of the automatic response. You may want to limit your telephone contact if it is difficult for you. Now that you are an adult, your primary caring must be directed toward your own well-being.

This exercise may be transposed to interviews for a job or to times set aside to meet with other people concerning a specific issue. For many of us, the cognitive (what we think) is aimed and fired properly, but the emotive (what we feel) creeps in to create confusion. One way to prevent such emotional turmoil is to rehearse, to write and to pre-experience what will take place.

PRESCRIPTION: FEELINGS

One of the areas where we may have some identifying to do is the "feelings" area. For various reasons, many adults have difficulty recognizing feelings and naming them. We know "good" or "bad" and nothing much else in between. Here is a list of some of the feelings that we may experience. How familiar are you with them? Have you ever experienced them?

abandoned	adamant	adequate	affectionate
agonized	almighty	ambivalent	angry
annoyed	anxious	apathetic	astounded
awed	bad	beautiful	betrayed
bitter	blissful	bold	bored
brave	burdened	calm	capable
captivated	challenged	charmed	cheated
cheerful	childish	clever	combative
competitive	condemned	confused	conspicuous
contented	contrite	cruel	crushed
culpable	deceitful	defeated	defiant
delighted	desirous	despair	destructive
determined	different	diminished	discontented
distracted	distraught	disturbed	divided
dominated	dubious	eager	ecstatic
electrified	empty	enchanted	energetic
enervated	enraged	envious	excited
exhausted	fascinated	fearful	flustered
foolish	frantic	frightened	free
frustrated	full	furious	gay
glad	groovy	guilty	gullible
happy	heavenly	helpful	helpless
high	homesick	honored	horrible
hurt	hysterical	ignored	immortal
imposed upon	impressed	infatuated	infuriated
inspired	intimidated	isolated	jealous
joyous	jumpy	keen	kind
kinky	laconic	lazy	lean
lecherous	left out	licentious	lonely
loving	low	lustful	mad

maudlin

melancholy

miserable

mystical

naughty

nervous

nice

niggardly

nutty

obnoxious

obsessed

odd

opposed

outraged

overwhelmed

pained

panicky

parsimonious

peaceful

persecuted

petrified

pitiful

pleasant

pleased

precarious

pressured

pretty

prim

prissy

proud

quarrelsome

queer

refreshed

rejected

relaxed

relieved

remorseful

restless

reverent

rewarded

righteous

ruptured

sad

sated

satisfied

scared

screwed up

servile

settled

sexy

shocked

silly

skeptical

sneaky

solemn

sorrowful

spiteful

startled

stingy

stranded

stuffed

stunned

stupefied

stupid

suffering

sure

sympathetic

talkative

tempted

tenacious

tense

tentative

tenuous

terrible

terrified

threatened

thwarted

tired

trapped

troubled

ugly

uneasy

vehement

victimized

violent

vital

vulnerable

weepy

wicked

wonderful

worried

Prescription: Colors

Because we can become confused with so many feelings, especially when we may lack some identification mechanisms, we may experiment with colors.

Materials
various clothes or paper swatches of different color
a willing adult
a suitable amount of time, say five days
a recording sheet

Exercise

At different intervals throughout your day, log or write down what you are feeling. The colors will help you to select a feeling: for example, red might suggest power, or grey, depression. It does not matter which colors you translate into which feelings; what does matter is that you become acquainted with the various feelings that you experience. As you gradually become more in tune with your feeling self, you will be amazed at how widely your feelings range within the course of one day. Some people will dress according to their feelings, to enhance them, or to eradicate them. Perhaps wearing a yellow t-shirt will chase away your down feelings, or a royal blue suit will dissipate your fearful feelings. You can experiment with feelings and know that they are indicators of how you experience life. There are no good feelings, no bad feelings, no feelings that you should not have. FEELINGS SIMPLY ARE. By acknowledging them, we can lessen their influence on our mood and enhance our behavior, without being ruled by them. I can *feel* angry without *doing* angry.

RECOMMENDED RESOURCES

1. Beavers, Robert. *Successful Families,*
   W.W. Norton & Company, New York, 1990
2. Bradshaw, John. *Creating Love,*
   Bantam Books, New York, 1992
3. ———. *Healing the Shame that Binds You,*
   Health Communications Inc, Florida, 1988
4. ———. *Homecoming*
   Bantam Books, New York, 1990
5. Jampolsky, Gerald. *Good-bye to Guilt,*
   Bantam Books, New York, 1985
6. Levin, Pamela. *Becoming the Way We Are,*
   Health Publications, Florida, 1988
7. McKay, Rogers and McKay. *When Anger Hurts,*
   New Harbinger Publications Inc, Oakland, 1992
8. Richardson, Ronald. *Birth Order and You,*
   Self-Counsel Press, North Vancouver, 1990
9. ———. *Family Ties that Bind,*
   Self-Counsel Press, North Vancouver, 1984
10. Weiser. *The Secret Lives of Snapshots and Albums*
    Brunner/Mazel, Vancouver, 1991

CHAPTER 3

REPARENTING

"Most kids hear what you say; some kids do what you say;
but all kids do what you do."
– K.C. Theisen

This chapter tells about a genesis. Where does one come from? What was mother like? What was father like? Our parents have affected us in various ways. Some of these ways are gifts that we want to cherish, preserve, and use in order to enhance our lives. Other influences that our parents have had on us might be a pattern we want to discard, or a memory we would like to heal. It is true for all of us that our parents did the best they could in parenting us; it is also true for all of us that, once we reach adulthood, we discover how their parenting was more or less effective. That's where we take our own parenting into our own hands and the "parenting of self" begins. The reflections and the exercises in this chapter on "reparenting" are not about parent-bashing. They are all about reconstruction, about reparenting ourselves: our adult ego can reparent our child ego.

Just as it is a difficult task to "re" do just about anything, so there is difficult work we can expect in reparenting ourselves. The amazing result lies in the fact that we discover our own parents, sometimes for the very first time, during the process of our own discovery of our true self.

CASE STUDY

Margaret presents herself as a calm, confident adult woman. Inside of her, there is something not quite right. Her friends, her family, and her colleagues have told Margaret that, once in a while, she becomes surprisingly distraught and frightened over the smallest of things. She becomes aware that she may have some unfinished business with her mother, since her anxiety seems to overtake her when her mother calls her unexpectedly.

When Margaret decides to seek out professional help, she wants to heal quickly. Her therapist tries to convey the message that it will take as long as it takes. The healing process is progressive as was the accumulation of pain that led her to therapy.

Some of the information that Margaret has about her family of origin is that her father died when she was three years old. She has no memory of him, except for photographs and stories that she has seen and heard. "Little

Maggie" and her mother lived for a few years with her maternal grand-parents, since her mother had a great deal of difficulty in coping with the death of Little Maggie's father. Later on in therapy, Margaret will confront her mother about her father's death, only to learn of the terror around his suicide.

Very gradually, Margaret uncovers many buried truths about her childhood: she lost a favorite cat when it was struck by a car, her mother suffered from depression while Little Maggie was growing up. Mostly, Margaret discovers that her inner child ego has never received much love, praise or positive reinforcement. Margaret begins her journey into reparenting with trepidation and a lot of hope.

EXERCISE IN SONG

The following exercise is based on the song, *Papa, Can You Hear Me?* It was recorded by Barbra Streisand (lyrics by M. Bergman). Listen to the recording and pay close attention to the words. There is also some therapeutic value in listening to the music as well, since it may evoke feelings within you that otherwise would remain suppressed.

This is a letter writing exercise. The aim is to communicate effectively with yourself on your relationship with your parents. It makes little difference whether or not they are living, whether or not your relationship with your parents was good or bad or a little of both. The processing of the letters may be done with a therapist, with a confidant, or with yourself alone. Some people do share these types of letters with their parents if they find it appropriate.

I suggest that you call your parents by their first names, such as Paul and Florence, especially if you have difficulty in conceptualizing them as human beings with their own limitations. This exercise may evoke feelings in you that have been repressed. Taking good care of yourself means checking to see how you experience the processing of this sort of letter. By all means seek professional help if you need to. You're worth it!

Dear

Your child

Prescription: Family Systems

What is a family system?

As mentioned in chapter two, a family system is a group of two or more persons, related by blood or by marriage. It is termed a "system" because the individual members organize automatically within it; each member influences the functioning of the entire system as well as each other. These are the dynamics of the system, that is, the way in which each member relates to the other. Factors such as individual temperaments, age, culture, religion, and sex will shape the dynamics of a family system.

What are parental roles?

The parents may be called the executive branch of the family system. Their role usually refers to their discipline or the way in which they establish their authority, either as a disciplinarian and rigid parent, as a wise and soft parent, as an aggressive parent or as a *laisser faire* parent who allows anything and everything.

What are family roles?

Some of the most common roles we find among the children of a family system are:
- The eldest – the responsible one.
- The baby – the spoiled one.
- The black sheep – the troublemaker.
- The quiet one – the one you never hear a peep out of, often a loner or lost child.
- The mascot – the entertainer, who enjoys clowning around.

What are the types of family systems?

The typical family systems are:
- Family of origin system – parents, children born of them, grandparents, uncles, aunts, cousins; consists of two or more generations.
- Blended family system – parents who have been married previously and divorced from their first partners, children may or may not be their biological children. It is the stepfamily system.
- Extended family system – includes the family of origin and the in-laws, as well as significant others, such as live-in nannies.

Note: For further reading on family systems, I recommend *Family Ties that Bind*, listed in the recommended readings.

Genogram Work

A genogram is really a visual duplication of our family of origin. We can use it to actually get a "picture" of our system. The following genogram of a family of origin is an example for you to follow.

Materials
some knowledge of names and dates
paper, pencil, colored markers

Symbols commonly used in genogram sketching
square for males
circle for females
diagonal lines for divorces
X for deceased persons
horizontal lines to partners
colors for various patterns of dysfunction such as alcoholism, workaholism,
    drug abuse; compulsive obesity, anorexia, bulimia; sex addiction; crimi-
    nal record; emotional, physical or sexual abuse; gambling; religious
    fanaticism; chronic illness, etc.
extensions for offspring of siblings
same extension line for twins
miscarriages and stillborns are marked with line extension and X

Sarah's Genogram

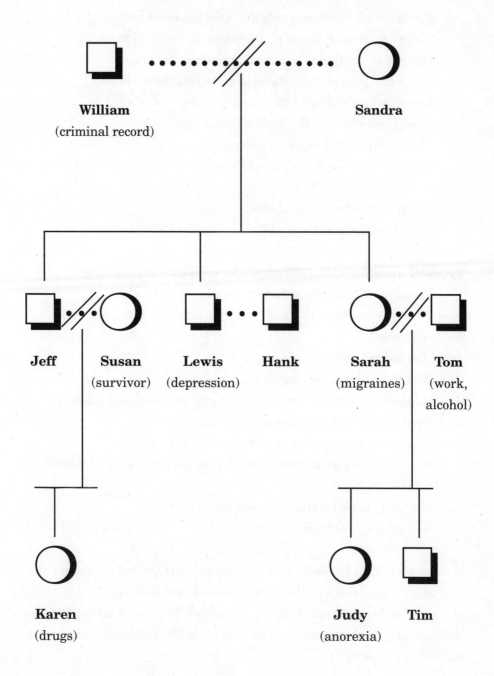

Sarah's genogram reveals the following information:

She is one of three children from a divorced couple.

She is the youngest and only girl with two older brothers.

There are three divorced relationships in her family of origin.

Her middle brother is in a homosexual relationship.

Sarah has two children, the eldest daughter is anorexic.

The oldest sibling's ex-wife is a sexual abuse survivor.

This oldest sibling's daughter is into drugs.

The middle sibling is a manic-depressive.

Sarah's ex-husband is a workaholic, and a heavy user, possibly abuser, of alcohol.

Sarah suffers from migraine headaches.

Sarah's father had a criminal record at one time.

Types of questions that Sarah might consider processing:

How did my father's past affect me when I was a child?

What was the unhealthiness of my parents' marriage, before the divorce?

How did that divorce affect me?

What type of relationship do I have with each of my siblings?

How did I experience being the only girl, the baby of the family?

What was my relationship like with Susan?

How do I experience Lewis's homosexual lifestyle?

What about my ex-partner? How did his workaholism and alcohol use affect me?

Why do I suspect Karen is into drugs?

How would I evaluate my mothering?

If you wish to find out more about genogram work, or build a more elaborate one, please consult the book *Genograms* in the recommended readings at the end of this chapter for further references. You may want to draw up a multi-generational genogram – very revealing. Recycling happens with or without our consent.

_____'S GENOGRAM

EXERCISE IN FILM

The following exercise is based on the film adaption of Neil Simon's play, *Lost in Yonkers*. Watching movies can be a very therapeutic exercise, if we have a purpose, something to look for, something to relate to. Often, from the experience of the characters, we can discover our own way of relating to others and to ourselves. The movie's characters can be mirrors of ourselves. I suggest you watch the film and do the exercise leisurely, giving yourself time and energy for introspection.

This is a "question and answer" exercise. Simply answer the questions in whichever way is comfortable for you. The intent is to get in touch with your family-of-origin system. Your responses might lead you to confide in someone, to seek sharing with a therapist or simply to keep, for your own awareness, any discoveries you make.

1. The grandmother did not like the boys' father. Why?

2. Describe the relationship between the boys and their father.

3. The grandmother is an interesting character, to say the least. How did she relate to her own sons, her daughter and her grandchildren? Which type of parental role did she play?

4. Bella is the daughter. Which role does she play in this family system? What is she all about? How does she relate to her siblings, to her nephews, to her mother?

5. Uncle Louis could be called the rebel, the black sheep, the different one. How does he relate to his mother, to his sister and his nephews? How has he "left home"?

6. As you reflect on your own family of origin and your role and place within it, have you become aware of anything specific from watching this film?

It is imperative to mention and to realize that all therapeutical exercises, and therapy on the whole, are progressive. Often, we become impatient and expect results as quickly as we can warm our soup in the microwave. There is no instant healing, no instant cure. Also, it is good to be aware that, sometimes, we will feel worse before we feel better. If a surgeon operates on you to remove your gall bladder, you can be sure that once the surgery is over, and once you awaken from the anesthetic, you will feel worse than when you were put to sleep. It will take a period of time before the surgical process will feel as if it's actually healing.

The same applies to healing from emotional wounds, or memories, or grieving issues; in fact, the same pattern applies to all therapeutical journeying. First there is a demolition stage, as I call it, when we stop the denial and get in touch with reality. This is followed by the confusion stage where nothing makes sense (during the stage of confusion, we also usually begin to get in touch with our emotions). Progressively we arrive at the last stage which is reconstruction. It is here that we face life, healed and accepting of what was, hopeful of what will be.

PRESCRIPTION:
WHERE OUR PARENTS COME FROM

It is important for us to have a sense of where our parents come from, and what it was like for them as children in their family of origin. Often, we come to know our uncles and aunts or grandparents only briefly; if we are fortunate, we become acquainted with them and keep a relationship lasting for many years into our adult life. The awareness of how our father and our mother experienced life when they grew up, helps to shed some light on our own patterns. Also, leading authorities, such as Minuchin and Bowen, believe that, in many ways, we live out our own experiences from our parents' perspective. Some psychotherapists will attest that we can even carry guilt, anger or sadness, as well as joy and a *joie de vivre* from a generation or two back. If this type of research interests you, please see the recommended readings at the end of this chapter.

The following questions are designed to help you become more aware of where your parents come from. Simply answer them as best you can. Research the answers if you prefer and share the process with a confidant or with a therapist, as you choose.

1. What role did each of your parents play in their family of origin? Eldest, youngest, lost in the middle, only child, responsible one, black sheep, mascot (the clown or entertainer of the family) or other designations you might find.

2. Complete the following statements as best you can.

    a) When my father was born, it was a time when...

    b) When my mother was born, it was a time when...

3. To the best of my knowledge, this is roughly the level of self-esteem that my parents had when I was born.

    (1 = poor; 10 = high)

    a) my father

    b) my mother

Some of you might be ready for a more pleasurable exercise by now. Here it is.

EXERCISE: GO SHOPPING

This pleasant exercise in reparenting brings back fond memories of a client of mine. John was in his early 60s when he came to therapy, to reparent himself; his father was emotionally absent in the family and his mother had pressured him to grow up quickly. I prescribed a shopping trip to the plaza, where he would buy himself some toys, some that he had wanted as a child but had not received. When he reported to me the following session, we had a chuckle over the way in which the store clerks observed him playing with the Tonka® trucks. Shopping for your child ego is quite therapeutic, as is playing, no matter how old you are. It's a bit of unfinished business that you as an adult might want to complete.

Materials

a willing adult

a suitable amount of funds

a desire to have a particular toy that one did not receive, but would have wanted as a child

Go shopping with your inner child.

After you have completed this shopping exercise, you may want to share it with a friend, a partner (it's great if the two are one and the same) or with a therapist. You might want to process the experience of a wish fulfilled and a sense of reparenting one's self. I wouldn't worry too much about the stuffy adults in the stores that will look at you with amusement; you can always tell them that Louise sent you.

EXERCISE: A SANTA LIST

I have used the following exercise several times with people who are into reparenting themselves; also, we use it in our home, so that everyone's child ego can join in the festivities.

Materials
a willing adult
a child ego
some wishes for a Santa list
    (they may be things, or ideas, whichever suits you)
Santa's address: SANTA CLAUS, NORTH POLE, H0H 0H0

_____'s Santa List

1.

2.

3.

4.

Do your best, Santa,

_____

Exercise:
Affirmations to Myself

This exercise stirs up fond memories of one of my clients. When this adult woman returned for a session, I had decorated my office with various affirmations about her: you can do it – I believe in you – I care about you – you are brave and courageous – etc. The impact of these affirmations on this client, with whom I was doing some reparenting work, was strong. Yet it is even better to be able to affirm ourselves than to have someone else affirm us. That is, the adult self affirms the child self, OR, reparents the child within us.

Materials
a willing adult self
a child self who needs some positive reinforcements
a tape recorder
a blank tape

Our own voice is also our signature; it can provide some sensory impact for our inner child thus reinforcing the parenting of oneself.

With a tape recorder, tape some positive reinforcing affirmations for your child self; use messages that you think might have been overlooked by your parents, messages that you think your child self could benefit from. Using your own adult voice to affirm yourself can be quite therapeutic. I suggest you repeat this exercise many times, whether in quiet times or while driving your car, whichever you can manage. With the repetition, your subconscious mind can register and also transmit to your conscious mind the affirmations as truths, which they are already. It is an exercise in convincing yourself that you are a lovable child and a lovable adult.

Prescription:
Petting Furry Creatures

I think it is wonderful that some institutions now have dogs or cats as residents. We know that the caring and the petting of animals has a therapeutic effect on those who are chronically ill or aging. There was a report in a recent publication about a quadriplegic woman who began to communicate with a dog; this was the first sign of communication that this woman had uttered in over five years. The tactile effect and the emotional effect of pets should be considered as an important tool in reparenting work. There is something very soothing in touching a dog or a cat, and an equally soothing experience in being licked by them. Also, their unconditional love and acceptance of who we are is powerful, especially for those of us who might have lived with conditions set, in order to be approved and loved.

Materials
a willing adult
a child self
a dog, or a cat, or any other animal that attracts you

Take time to sit with the pet. As you speak to them, gently stroke them. Allow the pet to touch you back. Enter into a relationship with this pet, if you can, whether it be visiting regularly or even better, adopting them into your family. You will be amazed at how the pet will communicate with you, how you will receive acceptance, and how you will experience validation from your pet.

Conclusion

Because this type of reparenting work has potential for emotional impact, I want to caution you about " self-help" groups. These groups are therapeutic if they are used with healthy boundary setting. Protect yourself from self-help groups that do not encourage closure, an end to the work. These will keep you stuck in the pain, in the memories; in fact, keep you dependent on the group itself. Because you want to heal, to go on, to leave the graveside, you will want to graduate at some point from the groups you choose to be involved with. It is very much like when we parent our children: we want to parent so that we can let our children take solo flight. If we do not prepare our children to leave home, then we have not done our work effectively.

You might want to give yourself a graduation party once you feel that you have achieved some form of healing. Personally, I enjoy a party every so often for the new things that I graduate from. Whether I celebrate myself for having had the courage to confront an old fear or whether I celebrate myself for not asking my father figure to approve of my decision, each celebration brings a renewed self.

Maybe your parents were too busy to effectively parent you, maybe they did not know how, maybe they were just too burdened with their own problems. Whatever the reason, it is unimportant. More than that, it is time to cease using your parents as an excuse. You can do the job. You can finish the job. You can reparent yourself.

RECOMMENDED RESOURCES

1. Black, Claudia. *It Will Never Happen to Me!*
   M.A.C. Publications, Denver Colorado, 1981
2. Blatner, Adam. *Art of Play: An Adult's Guide to Reclaiming Imagination*
   Human Sciences Press Inc., New York, NY, 1988
3. Bradshaw, John. *The Family*
   Health Communications Inc., Deerfield, 1988
4. Carnes, Patrick. *Don't Call It Love*
   Bantam Books, New York, NY
5. Framo, James. *Family of Origin Therapy*
   Brunner/Mazel Inc., New York,
6. Gordon, Thomas. *P.E.T. Parent Effectiveness Training*
   New American Library, New York
7. Kaminer, Wendy. *I'm Dysfunctional, You're Dysfunctional*
   Addison-Wesley Publishing Comp., Toronto, 1992
8. Marlin, Emily. *Genograms*
   Contemporary Books, Chicago, 1989
9. McFarland, Barbara. *Feeding the Empty Heart*
   Hazelden Foundation, Center City
10. Miller, Alice. *For Your Own Good*
    Collins Publishers, Toronto, ON
11. Napier, Nancy. *Recreating Your Self*
    W.W. Norton & Company, New York, 1990
12. Richardson, Ronald. *Birth Order and You*
    Self-Counsel Press, North Vancouver, 1990
13. ———. *Family Ties that Bind*
    Self-Counsel Press, North Vancouver, 1984
14. Secunda, Victoria. *Women and Their Fathers*
    Delacorte Press, New York 1992
15. Wegscheider-Cruse, Sharon. *Choicemaking*
    Health Communications, Inc., Florida, 1985

CHAPTER 4

INNER CHILD

"Problems cannot be solved with words, but only through experience, not merely corrective experience but through a reliving of early fear, sadness and anger."
— Alice Miller

This chapter encompasses various exercises and concepts concerning our adult lives, that part of our adult life that remains connected to our childhood life. Today we are aware of the deep effect that our childhood has on the way in which we live our adult life. As an adult, do I know how to play? Do I have unfinished business from my childhood that still haunts me? How did my family role affect me? Do I become frightened at certain events, in front of certain people and not understand where or why the fear comes over me? Do I experience life as a state of "alive bubbliness" or do I endure life as a sad and depressing space to be? How do I react and/or respond to childhood photos of me? How was I parented? How do I parent my children?

It is not by choice that our child self remains alive and acts out in our adult life; it is simply a fact. We know today that self-destructive patterns such as alcoholism, drug use or other forms of abuse to oneself are engineered by the child self: unhappy, frightened, angry or rebellious. After working through the first three chapters, you have some awareness of your childhood. Now the idea is to integrate the inner child into a wellness as an adult, so that our relationships with others and with ourselves are healthy.

CASE STUDY

Paula is a thirty-something professional woman. Her present problem is marital breakup. She reports needing to leave her relationship. According to her, her partner emotionally neglects her; there has been verbal abuse in the last several years; she has tried to bring her unhappiness to his attention.

When we begin to sketch her childhood history, we discover that she was the middle child, abandoned and left on her own a great deal; a lot of emotional neglect is apparent. At first, Paula is not sure why we need to look back but, as we progress, it becomes apparent to her that she has married a man very much like her older brother, who was a surrogate father. Her father was aloof, often absent from the lives of the family. As we go through a photo session, Paula begins to sob at the sight of the sad child that she was; in fact, she reports that this inner child of hers is very much alive and sad in this marriage.

Whenever her partner verbally puts her down, it is her mother's voice that she hears, saying that she cannot do such and such a thing. As we progress with experiential exercises in inner child work, Paula begins to rediscover her healthy child – the one who is curious, who explores, who laughs and who plays – in effect, the real inner child.

During our sessions, Paula visualizes that her inner child is probably three or four years old, and usually hiding behind a curtain when the adult Paula reaches out for her. We process this as signifying how a child reacts to the adult that seemingly abandoned it. It will take some time, some coaxing maybe, for the inner child to feel safe enough to come out and be vulnerable.

After a few months of intensive work, Paula left her relationship. She began to let go of her need for sleeping pills and anti-depressants, bought a shiny red sports car, and a Raggedy Ann doll. Now, once in a while, she takes her inner child for an ice cream cone and a ride on the swings in the park.

Exercise in Song

The chosen selection is titled *Tomorrow Child,* from the album *Playing to an Audience of One,* by David Soul. Listen to the song. Try to be aware of your own childhood, and the childhood of your children, if you have any.

This is a letter writing exercise. In order to capture the essence of the feeling of child self, try using your non-dominant hand to write this letter. You will discover more feeling connected to the content if you use this non-dominant hand. Perhaps you might share your experience with a confidant, a therapist, or a family member. What is important for you is the experience in your journey back and in your journey forward. This letter is from your child self, or your inner child, at age six, telling the adult you what it needs from you.

Dear Adult Me,

Your inner child,

Some people find it very rewarding to keep a journal with the inner child they discover. Each day, the child can write with the non-dominant hand how it experiences life with the adult self. The adult you can respond in the dominant hand to the inner child and progressively build a healthy relationship with the inner child. One thing is certain, whether or not we adopt our inner child and learn to live healthily with them, that child remains with us, an integral part of who we are forever.

EXERCISE IN FILM

Your inner child will be thrilled with the following selection, *The Velveteen Rabbit*; you may already know the classic story by Margery Williams. Either way, get out the popcorn and the soda and laugh along. Parts of this animated movie are for your adult self as well.

This is a writing exercise. Answer the following questions as best you can. They address issues such as parental care, relationship of children with their toys, and the healthy quality of childhood. Sometimes, in our adult life, we might experience feelings that have been buried for a long time; as a child we automatically suppressed these painful emotions. Triggers to these feelings can be such things as music, movies, phone calls, conversations or readings. When we are hit by a trigger we feel, as intensely if not more deeply, that the painful situation is happening all over again. If you have difficulty because of triggers or past pains, please seek professional help to do this work.

1. How was the child emotionally neglected by his parents?

2. Did the child have security during his illness? Did your inner child? What types of aftermath do you experience because of this?

3. There is a great deal of grieving for this child. Do you have grieving issues that need to be addressed? Did you lose a friend, a pet, a toy?

4. Observe and note the powerful relationship that develops between the fantasy friend and the boy. Did you have a make-believe friend? Do you now?

5. What do you suspect is the "real clockwork," that is, what makes him or her tick?

6. How is your inner child "real"?

The following exercises are instruments for use in inner child work, or inner child reclaiming. The basic principle is to get in touch with your inner child, to heal some of the childhood wounds that might represent unfinished business, and to get on with a quality of relationship between your adult self and your inner child self. The more remote and disengaged you are from your inner child, the more these exercises might seem bizarre or embarrassing to you; this could be an effective checkpoint for you, to evaluate just how in touch you are with this inner child part of you. Trust in the process. It works. It's never too late to have a happy childhood! If your childhood was happy, then you can celebrate those memories and integrate them into your daily living.

PRESCRIPTION:
ADOPT YOUR INNER CHILD

This is done by adopting a doll. Some of you might prefer a doll that you had as a child or a stuffed toy; what is imperative is that you feel drawn to the doll or to the toy. The concept of this adoption is for you to adopt your inner child. Once this is done, I recommend finding a special place in your home for your doll/inner child and make it a treasured part of your life and existence.

On the following page is a certificate of adoption for my inner child; you will notice it is in French since it is the language that my inner child speaks. I recommend allowing your inner child to reclaim their mother tongue as it proves more therapeutic. Your adult self will now parent your inner child. It is important that you acquire the doll yourself as opposed to receiving it from someone else. The principle of healthy individuation and of healthy boundaries is marked by this owning of one's own inner child.

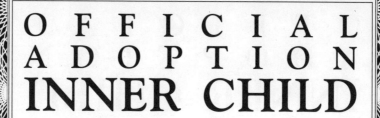

OFFICIAL ADOPTION
INNER CHILD

This certifies that the inner child

Petite Louise

was born on

le 28 mai 1951

with birthmark

un cœur sur la poitrine gauche

the official guardian

Louise Giroux

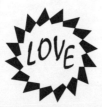

To acknowledge
To accept
To cherish
To protect

Louise Giroux (adult)

guardian

OFFICIAL
ADOPTION
INNER CHILD

This certifies that the inner child

_____

was born on

_____

with birthmark

_____

the official guardian

_____

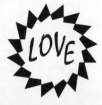

To acknowledge
To accept
To cherish
To protect _____

guardian

Prescription: Family Roles

The Characteristics, Traits, Feelings, Behaviors

ROLE	BEHAVIOR	FEELINGS	FOR FAMILY	LIABILITIES
Responsible	little mother, little man, does right, over achiever, over doer	hurt, inadequate, guilt, fear, low self-esteem, never enough	provides self-worth someone to be proud of	workaholic, never wrong, marries a dependent, manipulative, compulsive
Scapegoat	hostile, defiant, withdrawn, gets negative attention	hurt, alone, anger, rejection, low self-esteem	takes the focus off family problems	addictive trouble, lives on the edge
Lost	loner, dreamer, solitary, shy, ignored, drifts along	unimportant, lonely, defeated, abandoned	gives relief, the kid that the family never worries about	indecisive, no zest, little fun, alone or promiscuous never says "no"
Mascot	supercute, immature, hyperactive, short attention span	low self-esteem, inadequate	provides comic relief	compulsive, stressed, marries a hero, hysterical

Much of the role that we played as a child, and as a part of our family system, we maintain throughout our lives. Once we discover what that role is all about, we can be more aware of the liabilities that it can bring and channel into the assets that the role can encompass.

THE RESPONSIBLE ONE becomes competent, organized, responsible, and successful.

THE SCAPEGOAT displays courage and is good under pressure; usually helpful to others and not afraid of taking risks.

THE LOST CHILD, grown into an independent adult, is often talented, creative and imaginative.

THE MASCOT is a charming host, quick-witted with a splendid sense of humor.

These are the four commonly-referred-to roles within a family; you might identify some variations or some combinations of these four major roles in people.

EXERCISE: FAMILY ROLES

Materials
a clear concept of your siblings
photo of each sibling and of yourself
4 pieces of construction paper, each a different color

The exercise involves the following steps:
1. Place each photo on a board, or table or other hard surface.
2. Cut out symbols for each role category, perhaps a dozen for each category.
   e.g. 12 red circles for mascot, 12 yellow squares for responsible.
3. As you reflect on each member of your family, assign a color circle, or square, or other shape you have chosen to each member.
4. As you progress you should get a clearer visual display of the roles in your family.
5. You might want to pay special attention to your own role in your family, in the past, the present, and its effects on you, both positive and negative.

Note: It should be noted that we may develop various roles as the family grows, as persons leave or enter into the system. Also, no role is cast permanently. We always have the option of changing it if we choose to do so, even if the family as a unit finds this disconcerting.

PRESCRIPTION: VISUALIZATION

The aim of this visualization is to gain a clear sense of how healthy children live in the world. We can learn from them and mostly we can enter into meaningful relationship with our inner child. This practice will provide you with rich information on what is missing in your life, in order to make it whole and integrated. Don't be afraid to repeat the visualization process to gain quick access to that part of who you are.

EXERCISE: BECOME ACQUAINTED WITH YOUR INNER CHILD

Materials
a willing adult
a comfortable, peaceful and safe environment
instrumental music if it does not distract you (suggestions in references)
an idea of how your perfectly happy and healthy inner child looks

To enter into relationship with your inner child, you may use the following visualization or you may tape your own adult voice, which is recommended. Because I am a woman, my inner child is a little girl and I have used the feminine pronoun. Picture your inner child as female or male as appropriate.

Take a deep breath...
in through your nose...
out through your mouth...
Again, counting backwards from ten to one as you exhale.
Relax and be certain that you are at peace and safe with your universe.
Allow your healthy and joyous inner child to enter into your mind's eye...
What is she wearing...
how is her face... her eyes... her hair... her hands...
What is she doing... what is around her... beside her...
Are there any sounds she hears... any smells to this beautiful joyous place...
What does your inner child taste....

Get close to her so that you can hear her speak to you...
Ask her how she comes to be happy... what makes her happy...
what is the secret of her lightheartedness...
Which skills has she acquired to be happy...
How has she learned to expect the good...
How does she see the world that surrounds her....

Listen to her for as long as she speaks to you... hear what she says...
her recipes for a childlike joy of living...
Very slowly, take her hand...
Lead her into your adult world with you...
heed the words she has spoken to you...
remember her recipe for living in happiness and contentment...
Take her into your world...

When you are finished, repeat the breathing exercise until you are ready to
return to the pre-visualization state.

Exercise: Creating Safety

Many of us remember being tucked in by a parent. The blankets were lovingly tucked under our feet, our favorite plush toy friend was handed to us
and most of all a soft loving kiss was placed on our forehead as we heard,
"Sweet dreams precious." If we have not experienced it, we can claim this
wonderful feeling of security. The inner child within us needs to feel safe
and protected, especially when certain events or certain persons enter into
our world and space.

Materials
a willing adult self
an inner child self
a doll or toy that represents your inner child
a stressful or frightening situation

The best way to describe this exercise is to relate how one client used it. She noticed that each time she was in the presence of her former spouse, her inner child took over and she became frightened. He could verbally abuse her and her adult self could not defend the inner child because the inner child was terrified of his anger, and the adult self had lost power to the child. The adult woman began to tuck her inner child safely in her bed with her favorite teddy bear, before she needed to speak or be in the presence of the man. The adult woman would verbalize to her inner child something like: "You stay here and have a nice nap. I will meet with him and defend you so that you remain safe here. You are too frightened to come along."

Perhaps you have noticed your inner child taking over while you are on the telephone; if your child fears authority you will notice what transpires when you allow her to be part of a conversation where an authority figure and yourself are in contact. Your racing heart, your rushing blood, your sweaty palms and maybe that knot in your stomach are all indications that your inner child is frightened and needs to be protected by your adult self. The more you become familiar with your patterns, the easier it will be for you to do this exercise and to champion your inner child.

Exercise: Lego®

Somewhere around the age of two or three, we became aware that there were other children similar to us in our world. This was the beginning of our socialization phase; it became so much more interesting to play with other children than to play alone. The following exercise will be an effective way to discover how you relate to others, how you interact with peers. In order to do this exercise, you will need to invite four other adults who are willing to play along. If possible these adults should have some notion of inner child self, since the exercise suggests that we play as children.

Materials
five willing adults
five inner children
a good selection (about 500 pieces) of Lego

The participants sit together in a circle with the Lego strewn all over the floor in front of them. The task is to make one thing together, that is to build a common project together. Each member will not communicate verbally to the others or touch the others. All communication must be done by facial expression. Allow yourselves about 30 minutes of creative time to build the project. The product or the art created with the Lego is purely irrelevant. What matters is the way in which you participate in this group and what happens to you as you are active in the group, or inactive and passive, whatever the case may be for you. Once you have done the exercise, you can process with the other members the types of patterns that you experienced. Here are a few suggestions for how you can process this together:

• Did you experience different feelings during the course of the activity?
• Which feeling was most prominent for you?
• Did you experience any frustration, anger, or jealousy?
• Who led the group?
• What was your role: leader, caretaker, mascot, scapegoat?
• How was this a facsimile of relational patterns?

RECOMMENDED RESOURCES

1. Berenstain, Stan and Jan Berenstain. *The Berenstain Bears and The Bad Dream*
   Random House of Canada Ltd., Toronto, 1988
2. Dinkmeyer, Don. *Parent's Handbook (The)*
   American Guidance Service, Circle Pines
3. Ephron, Delia. *How to Eat Like a Child*
   Penguin Books, New York, NY, 1988
4. Fulghum, Robert. *All I Really Need to Know I Learned in Kindergarten*
   Villard Books, New York, 1990
5. Gil, Eliana. *Outgrowing the Pain*
   Dell Publishing, New York
6. James and Jongeward. *Born to Win*
   Addison-Wesley Publishing Company, Don Mills, Ontario, 1976
7. Keating, Kathleen. *The Hug Therapy Book*
   CompCare Publications, 1983
8. Larsen, Ernie and Carol Larsen Hegarty. *Days of Healing, Days of Joy*
   Hazelden Foundation, 1987
9. Levine, Pamela. *The Fuzzy Frequency*
   Trans Pubs, San Francisco, 1978
10. McConnell, Patty. *A Workbook for Healing*
    Harper and Row, San Francisco, 1983
11. Miller, Joy and Marianne Ripper. *Following the Yellow Brick Road*
    Health Communications Inc., Florida, 1988
12. Minuchin, Salvador. *Family Therapy Techniques*
    Harvard University Press, Cambridge, 1981
13. Pressman, Barbara. *Family Violence; Origin and Treatment*
    Children's Aid Society, Guelph, ON, 1987
14. Saint-Exupéry, Antoine. *The Little Prince*
    Harcourt Brace Jovanovich Publishers, New York, 1943
15. Short, Robert. *The Parables of Peanuts*
    Fawcett World Library, NY, 1968
16. Tessmer, Kathryn. *Breaking the Silence*
    A.C.A.T. Press, Santa Rosa, CA, 1986
17. Williams, Margery. *The Velveteen Rabbit*
    Running Press, Philadelphia, PA, 1981

CHAPTER 5

SEXUALITY

"Sex is a foretaste of the world to come."
– Talmud Brachot 57-B

This chapter deals with sexuality in its widest sense, that is, much more than sexual activity, preference, or energy, it encompasses all that makes a person a sexual being. How comfortable are you with your sexual identity? Were your role models, usually your parents, healthy in their sexuality? How did their experiences influence you in yours? Do you suspect or know for certain if you were sexually abused? How clear is your sense of boundaries? What about your body image? Can you celebrate being a woman or a man?

This area is one in which a great number of people need to reflect, to come to terms with reality and to recycle their beliefs and their practices. Because of several sociological, religious and psychological variants, sexuality is an area of continuous recycling in which one can experience turmoil as well as taste the sweet nectar of humanness.

Recycling means redefining, making from old material, beginning again. This is not intended to disregard who we were or what we had prior to this time. We find our past, meet with the key figures, relive childhood experiences, either through imagination or therapy. We then select the recyclable, the strengths, the good, the salvageable and we create a new life. There is no getting away from where we come from, who we were as a child, so why not glean everything positive we can from that part of our lives.

Recycling is learning about how we function in relationships, what our shortcomings tend to be and how our strengths can bring gratifying love into our lives.

CASE STUDY

Roger is a middle-aged man, very charming; he immediately uses his womanizer charms on his female therapist. Luckily, she sees right through him and begins asking him about his sex history. This investigation leads to discoveries that his parents did not relate healthily in their sex life. His father was promiscuous and believed that women were created for sexual pleasure, men's pleasure that is. His mother had excessive puritan tendencies; she believed females to be evil temptresses of men.

As a child, Roger had not been hugged or kissed; he grew up with no sense of affection and believed it to be synonymous to sex. He thought that his penis was affection enough. No wonder his sex partners complained about his lack of tenderness. Because he had to wear tight fitting clothes, Roger grew up to dislike anything tight on him; the clothes he wore were usually unfashionable because he lacked knowledge in the art of dressing appropriately. As an unattractive and overweight teenager, he had suffered extremely low self-esteem; his body was repulsive to him; therefore he concluded that it was repulsive to every person who saw him.

At a young age, Roger had ventured to a prostitute in order to check out what this sex stuff was all about. His loss of virginity to her disappointed him and this experience led to more of the same: no affection, simply sexual release. In his first marriage, Roger had been a very demanding sexual partner, one who hurried through sex while his partner endured it; of course, he had selected a partner who accepted this type of sexual abuse.

Soon after, Roger began to re-enact what his father had done and became promiscuous. Each and every sexual escapade drew him farther down into greater self-loathing. It was at this point of depression that he entered therapy and began the long process of recycling and reclaiming his sexuality. The treatment was to adopt a healthy sense of his identity, to discard his parents' messages on the subject of sexuality and to begin anew in his experience of sex. To learn about affection was a painful process because he needed to allow someone else to see his vulnerability; affection without sex became a new and thrilling adventure for him. Slowly, he learned to dress fashionably yet comfortably. After months of arduous work, Roger did marry for a second time; this time he experienced an almost virginal sexual experience, an authentic honeymoon and an indescribable sense of healthy sexuality.

EXERCISE IN SONG

The chosen selection is titled *The Power of Love*, recorded recently by Céline Dion. As you listen to the recording, try to become aware of the feelings that it evokes within you. This song speaks of a loving and healthy intimacy between two people.

This is a writing exercise. The intent is for you to write to a partner; you may select a spouse, a former lover, a current lover. After hearing and thinking about the song, you probably have some sense of your intimacy level with this person. Write him or her a letter in which you can share this part of your sexuality with them.

My dearest lover,

Your loving partner,

EXERCISE IN FILM

The following is another exercise in cinematherapy. For this chapter, I recommend two films. The first is the well-acclaimed, *Fried Green Tomatoes* and the second is *A River Runs Through It*. We will focus on women's issues in the first and men's issues in the second. It would be ideal for you to take time to view both films since we all need more awareness of the sexuality and other challenging life issues of the opposite sex.

Fried Green Tomatoes: women's sexuality and women's issues

The first film is *Fried Green Tomatoes*. The intent is for you to focus on the four female characters in the story: Mrs. Threadgood (the octogenarian), Evelyn, Ruth and Idgy (the young Mrs. Threadgood). These four women represent life at various stages; they offer a quality cross-section of women's sexuality and women's issues.

Women: Four portraits

The following questions will help to direct your awareness to the four different portraits of these women. In doing so, you will have the opportunity to get in touch with various issues concerning sexuality.

IDGY

What is her "type" of woman?

As a young girl, what was her socialization like?

Who was her male role model and how did this affect her?

How is she a liberated woman from her social period?

RUTH

How does she own her sexuality?

She functions for some time as a victim. How?

Which elements free her from abuse?

How is she the "perfect lady" type?

MRS. THREADGOOD

What is the theme of her conversation?

How does her hair color affect her behavior?

Why and how is she a model for Evelyn?

What about her mothering skills?

What parts of the young Idgy has she maintained into octogenarianism?

EVELYN

What do you suspect is her reason for eating chocolate bars and doughnuts?

Could she look at her vagina in a mirror?

How does she react to masturbation?

Does her husband contribute to her turmoil?

Does "the change" affect her? How?

What is the symbolism of slamming into the parked car?

Her anger, her acting out are factors in her liberation. How?

Which transitions has she lived through from the beginning to the end of the story?

ME (or MY PARTNER)

A River Runs Through It: **men's sexuality and men's issues**

The following questions and comparisons will help to direct your awareness to the male characters in this movie. In doing so, you will have the
opportunity to get in touch with various issues concerning male sexuality.

COMPARISON OF THE MACLEAN BROTHERS

	NORMAN	PAUL
1. General disposition and personality.		
2. How each interacts in social settings.		
3. Their relationship with their father.		
4. Their life ambitions.		
5. Their relationship with women.		

THE REVEREND MACLEAN

1. Which kind of parenting did Reverend Maclean use towards his sons?

2. Was he a feeling man, a thinking man, an aggressive man, or...?

3. Do you believe that he played a part in his sons' development of their own sexuality? How?

QUOTATIONS
Explain the following, from the film

1. "If boyhood questions aren't answered at the time, then they can never be answered again." (Norman)

2. "Education was a revelation." (Norman)

3. "The body fuels the mind." (Father)

4. "In Montana, the three things we're never late for are work, church and fishing." (Paul)

5. "Why is it that the people who most need the help won't take it?" (Jessie)

6. "Life is not a work of art, and the moment cannot last." (Norman)

7. "It is those we live with who elude us, but we can still love them without complete understanding." (Father)

8. "Eventually all things merge into one, and a river runs through it." (Norman)

GENERAL QUESTIONS

1. In the scene that Norman coins, "Macleans Conquer Chutes," the brothers, now young men, survive the rapids. Do you see any symbolism in this episode?

2. Norman narrates how his brother Paul developed an artistic way of fly fishing; he called it, "shadow casting." How does this part of Paul's life give us an insight into his character, his behavior and his death?

3. Neil, Jessie's brother, is presented briefly. What could you say about his character and his sexuality?

Prescription: Sex and Food

Planet Eros

Sex versus Food: Why the Difference?

It was late in the 22nd century when the starship Blintx first visited the galaxy containing the planet Eros. The people there were found to be surprisingly like those on Earth. The most unexpected difference was that their attitudes about sex and food were found to be the reverse of Earth's.

On Eros, sexual activity was totally accepted as a natural bodily function and as a source of pleasure to be cultivated by those with imagination and good taste. Children observed the sexual behavior of others from their earliest years and were encouraged to enjoy their bodies. Young people freely engaged in sexual games and naturally imitated the behavior of adults.

As a matter of course, movies, plays and T.V. shows contained explicit sexual scenes. On educational T.V. a middle-aged lady had a popular show that taught advanced sexual techniques and variations. There were also illustrated sex books containing "recipes" for special treats. Because of the central role that sexuality played in the lives of Erosians, they frequently sought entertainment or celebrated special occasions by going to public establishments called sexaurants, where both males and females were sexually served by courteous employees who worked primarily for tips. Many of these establishments were decorated to provide a special atmosphere (a particular ethnic subculture, a ship, a barn, and so forth) and the more opulent charged outrageously high prices. A few were made to revolve slowly on the top floor of tall buildings, thus providing a spectacular view of the city below while the patrons engaged in sexual pleasures. Much more economical establishments also were seen in each town – fast sex franchises that provided the basic sexual gratifications but dispensed with the fancy frills.

In this free and easy sexual atmosphere, the astronauts from Earth were amazed to find a very different reaction to food. Almost no one was willing to talk about his or her eating habits, and some blushed when the topic was mentioned. It seemed that everyone acknowledged that eating was a physical necessity, but it was very bad manners to talk about engaging in that behavior or – even worse – enjoying it. There were a few gender differences, and some females reported that they never had enjoyed a meal in their lives.

It was traditional to eat alone or in pairs in darkened rooms. There was a strong taboo against being seen eating or seeing anyone else eat. Occasionally, a deviant was arrested for peeping in a dining room window. Children were taught very little about the whole process; if a child was caught putting food in his or her mouth publicly, the child was warned that such practices will grow hair on their tongue, rot their brain, and cause blindness.

Nice people did not use four-letter words such as "fork" or "chew." No one was permitted to write about eating unless it could be shown that the total work had some socially redeeming value and was not designed simply to make people hungry. There were illegal novels and magazines that dealt with food, but many believed that hard-core material would cause people to run wild in the streets, committing unspeakable food crimes. Even worse were the rundown movie theaters in the larger cities that presented 16 mm films of people consuming an eight-course meal; the mostly male audiences sat quietly watching these scenes while chewing gum.

In adulthood, it was expected that each person would begin to take meals only with a spouse, though it was known that some people had admitted sharing a snack or two with someone else's mate. There were a few shady establishments where they sometimes went to order a gourmet meal prepared by a sordid young lady.

In the more progressive communities, there were food-education courses in the schools; these were taught to sexually segregated classes and dealt primarily with the technical details of digestion plus sections on the dangers of obesity and food poisoning. There was no indication in such courses that eating could be fun. The students sometimes drew crude pictures on the walls of the eating cubicles showing people eating. There were messages such as "Mary likes squash" followed by a telephone number.

Eros seemed strange to the visitors from Earth, and vice versa.

Author unknown

Now that you have read the story, consider the ways in which our society responds differently to the biological needs for food and for sex. Why do you think there are such differences? Could there really ever be a society such as the one on Eros? Basing your conjectures on what is known about the way sexual attitudes and beliefs are learned, try to determine how food-related attitudes and beliefs would be learned on this imaginary planet.

EXERCISE:
REFLECTION OF MY BODY

Materials
a mirror, preferably full length
a willing adult
no clothes

This exercise is by no means an original. It has been recommended for many people including Evelyn in *Fried Green Tomatoes* in her "sexuality" group. With all the media hype on body image, women and men have been pressured to look for the "perfect" body–the *Cosmo* model type or the "sexy is thin" type. I've always thought it was a shame that I did not live in the Rubenesque period when I would have been the envy of all women and the desire of men with my large breasts and wide behind! Well, back to the exercise.

- Take all the time you need, the idea is to do this daily for a few seconds rather than for long periods at a time.
- Stand in front of a mirror and observe one part of your body – one eyebrow, one lip, a cheek, nose, two fingers, etc.
- As you observe that part of your anatomy, be willing to accept it as your temple, who you are – not how you would prefer it to be – but as you are now.
- Do not connect with the same part twice, so that eventually you will deal with each part of your body.
- Take note of the health in your body, of what each part of you does for your organism.
- Be aware of the parts that need special care from you and be willing to care for them.

- It is important to connect with your genitalia, to accept this part of who you are, this part of you that offers pleasure to you.
- As you do this exercise, touch yourself gently and with care, as you would someone you truly love and respect; your body needs affection from you also.
- If you notice that a certain part of your body needs medical attention, take care of it.

You could finish the exercise by taking a warm bubble bath, by relaxing your muscles and your other metabolical systems. Congratulate yourself even if you have difficulty in doing the exercise at first and be assured that each few minutes will gradually work into time spent therapeutically with your own temple.

EXERCISE:
WOW!! I CAN DO THAT!!!

One area of sexuality that is often repressed due to cultural, religious, and social factors is our capacity for orgasm. Our first experience with being orgasmic is, unfortunately, often a frightening mystery, especially if we are involved in an activity that is taboo. For both women and men, that first encounter with masturbation or with a sexual partner, when we become aware of our body's wondrous capacity for orgasm, is often welcomed with shame or guilt and very seldom with celebration. It just isn't the type of thing we run out into the living room to announce to our parents, "Guess what I just did?" We usually leave this sort of communal celebration for report cards. Now that we are adults and have a clear sense of private and intimate boundaries, we can celebrate this part of us. I am advocating a private time, as I believe sexual activity to be private, in which we can accept and appreciate our own sexuality.

PRESCRIPTION:
CELEBRATING MENSES

The intent of this piece on menstruation is to offer some time to reflect and to become fully aware of this area of our sexuality. It involves our partners as much as it does us, since we share a life in which there is this element of variability brought on by our cyclical dimension.

In my personal experience and in the experience of many women of my generation, most of us learned about menstruation and women's cyclical patterns, as well as men's hormonal times and cyclical patterns, from word of mouth and unfortunately not always knowledgeable mouths. When we take time to reflect, menstruation is one of the most precious gifts that personkind has – the ability to make new life. As you read the following excerpt from Steinem, have a good chuckle as well as some thought on how your menstruation or your partner's menstruation affects your lives.

"If Men Could Menstruate..."
What would happen, for instance, if suddenly, magically, men could menstruate and women could not? The answer is clear – menstruation would become an enviable, boast-worthy, masculine event:

Men would brag about how long and how much.

Boys would mark the onset of menses, that longed-for proof of manhood, with religious ritual and stag parties.

Sanitary supplies would be federally funded and free. (Of course, some men would still pay for the prestige of commercial brands such as John Wayne tampons, Muhammad Ali's Rope-a-dope pads, Joe Namath Jock Shields – "For those light bachelor days," and Robert "Baretta" Blake Maxi-Pads.)

Gloria Steinem, "If Men Could Menstruate," *Ms. Magazine,* October 1978.

EXERCISE

This is a writing exercise. Write a letter to your partner in which you will address your needs and your gratitude for his or her participation in the cyclical patterns of your life. Share the letter with the person and agree to stay connected on this issue.

Dear

Your loving partner,

PRESCRIPTION:
PROTECTING MY BOUNDARIES

Our boundaries are the psychological, the emotional and the physical surroundings we create to protect ourselves from outer harm. For instance, we
will say that a person's physical boundaries are violated when they are hit
by someone else; that a person's sexual boundaries are violated when they
are fondled involuntarily by someone else; that being verbally put down is a
violation of emotional boundaries.

We develop our sense of boundaries and remain responsible for their safety
at an early age; this is why we now have school programs to teach children
to recognize when someone violates their boundaries. If our parents or
parent figures invaded our boundaries consistently, either by verbally, emotionally, physically or sexually invading our private space, then we may
have grown to have an unclear and undetermined sense of protection of our
boundaries. We probably cannot say "no" easily, cannot ask for the visitor to
return at a more appropriate time, cannot confront the person who verbally
puts us down.

Boundaries are nebulous, intangible. Only when we have begun to establish our own system of boundaries and have tasted the positive feeling of
challenging those who invade ours, can we truly be aware of the sacredness
of boundaries.

EXERCISE

This exercise consists of a fictitious invasion of boundaries; it is better per-
formed with someone who has a sense of boundaries and of what we are
doing.

Materials
a willing adult
another willing adult to partake in the exercise
a box of tissues, rolled into individual balls

Your partner in the exercise will gently throw the balls of tissue towards you, one at a time, from various directions. As each tissue approaches your boundary, you will gently tap it, thus causing it to fall to the floor, not entering into your private space.

The intent is to disallow any type of interference from the outside when you choose to safeguard your boundaries. As you progress in the exercise, imagine that each tissue transforms into a person verbalizing or a figure confronting or words being uttered – whatever types of imaginings could be violating your boundaries.

Just as we protect our own boundaries, we are responsible to safeguard others' boundaries. Because our partner is intimate with us, does not give us a license to invade his or her boundaries. Respect is the key word here and healthy love is the optimum.

You will find it fascinating to observe how others usually exhibit the same type of boundary restrictions that you do, once you are aware of your own and once you claim those as your own. Depending on whether you and your partner are introverted or extroverted, you will need to communicate about which types of boundary settings are appropriate for both of you. When they differ, you can simply negotiate to respect each other's patterns.

RECIPE FOR HEALTHY SEXUALITY

Ingredients
well-ripened adults
candles, fragrance, bubble bath
sensual lingerie or nudity
soft music
grapes or strawberries
massage oil
open and healthy attitude
private space, doors locked

Process

Mix all of the ingredients together, very slowly, as to keep the unique flavor of each.

Make sure the atmosphere is right, all of the senses being used by the participants.

Use verbal skills at random when it is comfortable to do so.

Erase old ideas of negativity concerning sexuality.

Enjoy the moment.

RECOMMENDED RESOURCES

1. Cohen, Betsy. *The Snow White Syndrome*
   Jove Books, New York, 1986
2. Comfort, Alex, Editor. *More Joy of Sex*
   Pocket Books, Toronto, ON, 1973
3. Fezler, William and Eleanor S. Field. *The Good Girl Syndrome*
   Macmillan Publishing Ltd., New York, 1985
4. Friday, Nancy. *My Secret Garden*
   Pocket Books, New York, 1973
5. ———. *Forbidden Flowers*
   Pocket Books, New York, 1975
6. ———. *My Mother / My Self*
   Pocket Books, New York, 1972
7. ———. *Jealousy*
   A Perigord Press Book, New York, 1985
8. ———. *Women on Top*
   Pocket Books, New York, 1991
9. Frisch, Melvin. *Stay Cool through Menopause*
   The Body Press, New York 1993
10. Hirschman, Jane and Carol Munter. *Overcoming Overeating*
    Fawcett Columbine, New York, 1988
11. Minirth, Frank. *Love Hunger*
    Fawcett Columbine, New York, 1990
12. Orbach, Susie. *Fat Is a Feminist Issue*
    Berkley Books, New York, 1978
13. Powter, Susan. *Stop the Insanity*
    Simon and Schuster, New York, 1993
14. Secunda, Victoria. *Women and Their Fathers*
    Delacorte Press, New York, 1992
15. Simmons, Richard. *Never Give Up*
    Warner Books, New York, 1993
16. Steinem, Gloria. *Revolution from Within*
    Little Brown Company, New York, 1992
17. Taylor, Elizabeth. *Elizabeth Takes Off*
    G.P. Putnam's Sons, New York, 1987

CHAPTER 6

COUPLE

RELATIONSHIPS

"Partners have been communicating for thousands of years with a caring spirit. No substitute exists for love and caring in communication! However, even with a caring attitude, communication can be unclear, inept, or misunderstood. This is where skills enter."
– *Miller,* Talking and Listening Together

The ability to form relationships is a skill that we develop over a period of time. It is not something that is a given, that we acquire upon falling in love, but rather, a construction of day-to-day happenings, done in partnership.

Have you ever considered your life without a partner? How do you view your level of interdependency with another? Although you may verbalize well, do you listen as intently as you speak? Are sexual issues discussed openly between you and your partner? Which is your type of personality: outgoing or withdrawn, attentive to detail or preferring the general picture, thinking rather than feeling? How does your personality affect your relationship? Because it is assumed that there are various stages or phases in a relationship, do you notice any difference in yours over the last few years? How does your family of origin and that of your partner affect your own relationship? What sorts of dance steps do you and your partner do in "interpersonal dance," that is, how do you relate and move closer to or away from each other? Do you step on each other's feet, or dance intimately close, or dance one in each corner of the room? These are some of the questions and topics that will be addressed in this chapter.

CASE STUDY

Mary and Tom are a middle-aged couple; they have requested marriage counseling. This couple have been married for 23 years, have three children, the youngest now being in high school. Upon assessment, it is clear that their communication is ineffective.

She speaks a great deal but without any acknowledgment of feelings; it is very easy to detect her pattern of control over her husband and her children. He says very few words and seems to be quite angry, probably into passive-aggressive mode; this means that he will withdraw his affection instead of confronting his partner. It is apparent that Mary does not listen to anyone; while the counselor speaks to her, she is busy coming up with a response or another instance of when Tom neglects her.

They have focused their relationship on their children, who were all born during the first five years of the partnership. Now that these children are independent, Mary complains of a void in her life, of how her husband is not a companion. Tom has no idea what that means since he has never been a companion. Their sex life is non-existent except for the rare times when, out of guilt, Mary seeks out Tom for sexual activity. He comes close to revealing that he is impotent because he has felt so inadequate in the shared couple activities.

Their relationship is bankrupt in terms of affection and of effective communication; they do not have the skills to share their world nor the skills to hear each other's sharing if it did occur. The therapist slowly points out to them that there is work to be done in communication; living with someone for a quarter of a century is not a guarantee that communication has taken place. Are they willing to do the work? Do they have the willingness to begin to forgive each other for whatever pain they caused the other? These patterns of relationship will be a challenge to break and the therapist informs the couple of this fact.

There were individual sessions in which each of the partners had a chance to get an overview of how they function in relationships. Each discovered how they react to being in a couple relationship, how they lead, how they function in a system. Also, they had the opportunity to see the effect of their family of origin roles in their marriage. Tom discovered that he had married a woman like his mother, very authoritative, a woman who controlled him. He even reacted the same way, by withdrawing into his repressed anger. Mary found that she had married a submissive man like her father, a fellow rather inclined to passivity, one she could control. Now they both understood that it would not work any longer and things needed to change.

The changes for Tom were liberating: he began to take his own voice, to refuse to do certain things and to strengthen his sense of boundaries. Mary found this very difficult and had a great deal of trouble in letting go of the control. She definitely lived in great fear of losing control and of somehow losing herself within this relationship.

After a few months, the couple decided to separate. Tom initiated this separation and he worked through it marvelously. For the first time in his life, he experienced independence and a happiness in being his own person. Unfortunately for Mary, she had a great deal of turmoil over the separation; her grieving was a desperate attempt at getting back what she thought had existed, although in reality it never had. Instead of the destruction of two people, the outcome was the pain of one who could not accept the changes and the release and peace of the other who actually turned his entire life around. Tom went on to be a man with the potential for healthy relationships.

EXERCISE IN SONG

The chosen song is one that was popular in the late '80s entitled *Flying on Your Own*, by Rita MacNeil. The intent of the exercise is to encourage you to tap into your own power, your own voice, sort of a solo-flight approach. It is not a condemnation of relationships in any way but rather a validation of and an invitation to self-dependency. More and more, we are becoming aware that one of the main factors in an unhealthy relationship is a weak or underdeveloped sense of self. After listening to the song, you might increase your awareness by doing the following writing exercise.

1. There are a few contrasts in these lyrics. How do they apply to your experience in relationships?

STRONG/ALONE

HAPPY/BLUE

WISE/FOOL

2. When you imagine yourself independent, alone, or in a relationship, how is this picture for you?

EXERCISE IN FILM

The film *Husbands and Wives*, directed by Woody Allen, presents an interesting account of the mechanics of relationships, how they function and what types of things make them break. I suggest that you watch about 20 minutes of the movie, do the recommended exercise, and then resume watching the movie. This will enable you to check out the accuracy of your "diagnoses" of the couple systems.

Gabe and Sally (Allen and Farrow)
What is your primary diagnosis of the problem in their couple system?

What is your tentative prognosis for this couple system?

Jack and Sally (friends)

What is your primary diagnosis of the problem in this couple system?

What is your tentative prognosis for this couple system?

After checking out your assumptions of these two couple systems, it might be interesting for you to do the same for your own couple system. Imagine that you and your partner are in a movie and outline what your system might be like.

Me and My Partner

What is the primary diagnosis of our system?

What is the tentative prognosis for our system?

PRESCRIPTION:
KNOW WHEN TO SEEK HELP

It is important to remember that these exercises are simply suggestions that allow for awareness and self-knowledge. If any or all of these create certain stresses in your life, I recommend that you seek professional help in order to deal with your issues. *How many marriages would be better if the husband and wife clearly understood that they are on the same side.*

EXERCISE:
PRESENTING MY PARTNER

The exercise consists of introducing your partner to a public of some sort. The presentation of him or her must be in positive terms only. In other words, by giving a very positive and accurate description of your partner, you accent the positive in your mate.

Here's _____

Let's hear it for _____

Prescription: Without You...

As you think about the future, also give some thought to how you would experience life without your partner. This will give you a clear indication of how independent you are, and how well you are individuated from your partner. If you are enmeshed, that is over involved with your mate, then you are experiencing what is known as codependence. Usually, in this sort of dynamic, both parties are inadequately able to function on their own, so what we have as a result is one half times one half, and the product of this multiplication is one quarter. What you want to strive for is a sum of two, that is, one whole person and one whole person.

In which areas would you need to promote your individuality? How is the fantasy of living without your partner for you? If the very thought throws you into a panic, you might consider doing more work in the area of independence. In the list of recommended readings, you will find resources dealing with techniques and approaches to living in *inter*-dependence as opposed to *co*-dependence. It's more a matter of completing one another than filling the voids in each other.

Exercise

The following exercise is to be done over coffee or tea, at the kitchen table or in the family room, anywhere other than in the bedroom; the idea being that it is much safer to discuss our sex life and sexuality in an area other than the one where we engage in the actual sexual activity. If you are fortunate enough to have been sexually active in all the rooms of your home, then go outside to discuss these questions. (You're kidding!!! On the front lawn too?)

Complete these sentence fragments, alternating between you and your partner.
What I like about the way you dress is...
What I dislike about the way you dress is...
I find my sex drive to be more... or less... than yours.
When you do not want to be sexual, I usually...

The frequency of our sexual activity is...

I am aware that before I was your sex partner, you...

So far, in the course of our relationship, our sex life has changed in that it...

My parents' sexuality and sex life has influenced me by...

The fact that our sexual activity is usually initiated by...

The idea of a perfect lover for me is one who...

If I were rating our sex life on a scale of 1 to 10...

In our overall life together, I think the importance of our sex is...

PRESCRIPTION: TEMPERAMENT TYPES

This section deals with psychological types or temperament types. First of all, you might want to read about the four major types which are sub-divided into two types each. The following is a summary of these types. More references are to be found in the recommended readings, particularly in *Connecting*, by Miller et al. or in *Please Understand Me* by Kiersey.

EXTROVERT OR INTROVERT
(Being oriented to the world)

Extrovert

turns outward to energize

talks, works, plays with others

moves quickly into action

likes to expend energy

too much aloneness is uncomfortable

Introvert

turns inward for renewed energy

finds inner world of ideas more important

contentment in reading

doing things alone is comfortable

looks for depth rather that breadth in relationships

may feel lonely in a crowd, seeks solitude

SENSING OR INTUITING
(Taking in information)

Sensing
concentrate on what they learn from the five basic senses
a detail-oriented person
one that emphasizes and trusts past actions

Intuiting
forms a general picture perception
may not seem to use information from the five basic senses
trusts hunches about the future

THINKING OR FEELING
(Coming to conclusions)

Thinking
analyzes and processes logically
looks at facts and principles
most conclusions are impersonal

Feeling
bases conclusions on degree of feeling
judges impact of decision on themselves and others
weighs what they like and dislike
conclusions may appear illogical

PERCEIVING OR JUDGING
(Dealing with the world/openness or closure)

Perceiving
is continually aware
desire for open-mindedness
may back away from decision, restless
may change their mind

Judging

comes to a conclusion, wants closure

wants order in their life

is outcome oriented

pushes for decisions and feels easy afterward

EXERCISE

This exercise consists of each individual member of the system, deciding on which types he or she is: either sensing or intuiting, either thinking or feeling, either perceiving or judging, either extrovert or introvert. Each person will have four components. Then, the couple can draw a chart to see which one of them fits where; finally how do these psychological types affect the relationship?

After you have observed the chart below which illustrates Bob and Carol's psychological types, answer the following question: How does this pattern of psychological types impact on the relationship between Bob and Carol?

EXTROVERT *Carol*	**INTROVERT** *Bob*
SENSING *Bob*	**INTUITING** *Carol*
THINKING *Bob Carol*	**FEELING**
PERCEIVING	**JUDGING** *Bob Carol*

In the first dimension, Carol is an extrovert while Bob is an introvert. Could this complement their dynamic? Could it cause conflict? Bob "senses" and Carol is "intuitive," yielding a complementary dynamic. Both partners are thinkers and neither is much into feeling. How could this create tension between them? Neither partner is perceptual but rather judging; could this be a source of conflict?

After observing the particular pattern of their couple system, you might consider your own pattern of relationship with reference to the temperament types. You will discover, if you do not already know, that no specific type or combination is "better" than the other; each has its weaknesses and its strengths. The key is to relate effectively with the pattern as it is established.

PRESCRIPTION:
IN-LAWS — MINE, YOURS, OURS

The wonderful world of in-laws is one that often brings challenge to a relationship. One reason for this is that a person may be accustomed to the pattern in their own family of origin, to the different members, and how to handle themself with the others. For their partner, however, this can be unknown territory and can develop into warfare. Indeed, couples who maintain healthy boundaries and enjoyment with their families of origin are very fortunate. As with every other area of therapeutic work, the key is to become aware and to touch our own experience of these people. Once we are made aware, we can then begin the task of making healthy our relationships within our respective families of origin.

Materials
two willing adults, in a relationship
family photos, family albums, various snapshots to represent members of the two families of origin
atmosphere of quiet exchange (not in the heat of an argument!)

EXERCISE

As both of you go through the various photographs, talk about the people you are seeing. How do you relate to them? What do they mean to you? Do you know them well or just slightly? This part of the exercise simply involves getting in touch with feelings around your families of origin.

Answer the following questions individually and then discuss your various answers with your partner.

1. How does my position in my family of origin affect my relationship with you? (eldest, youngest, middle...)

2. They say we marry a person like one of our parents. How are you like my father? How are you like my mother? What effect does this have on me?

3. In my sibling interaction, do I enhance or diminish the quality of our relationship?

4. Are there scenarios in my childhood that are repeated in our relationship? What is the effect on our relationship?

5. Does my parents' relationship affect my expectations of our relationship?

6. How does our relationship with our children perpetuate the patterns from our parents to us?

7. Which positive attributes of your family of origin would I like to carry into our life together?

Note: Allow yourselves a few minutes to talk about each answer. Contract to not go over the total time limit for the exercise. Often we go into discussion for too long a period of time, especially if the topic presents certain challenges. You and your partner probably have a sense of how much time you are comfortable with; remaining comfortable should be your priority. It is always easier to augment discussion time than it is to repair frustration over too much time spent.

PRESCRIPTION: SHALL WE DANCE?

As mentioned earlier, the way in which we relate and move towards and away from our partners is what is known as interpersonal dance. If you wish a complete study on this topic, read *Connecting* from the list of recommended resources. What is important to remember is that all couples dance together according to their own style of relationship. The following is a summary of the three patterns of interpersonal dance.

1st dance pattern: the "Glued together" dance
Positive

In this dance, the couple is open in its sharing; each one feels comfortable to joke around and to laugh or to cry and be vulnerable if need be. This sense of cohesion is usually found in newly formed relationships. There is no absence of touching; in fact, it is a continuous celebration of each other.

Negative

In this dance, the couple is in a constant state of conflict; whether through arguing, bickering, accusing or attacking, both persons are in a headlock. Each person is constantly defending her/himself as well as protecting her/himself from the other.

In the "Glued together" dance, the danger for both individuals is to experience a diminishment of their own identity. Less productivity outside the relationship may ensue. One danger is the potential for enmeshment, which usually manifests itself as overprotection or overinvolvement with the other.

2nd dance pattern: the "Breaking away" dance

In this dance pattern, one partner tries to influence the other. One will take the lead, trying to influence the other, whether it be in order to change a value, an interest, or a habit. How the second partner responds to the first's initiative determines whether or not something will change.

Positive

This dance can be positive when the new direction is supported and encouragement is verbalized. There is no resistance from the second partner.

Negative

This second partner may resist because he or she feels left out, or perhaps experiences the fear of becoming disconnected to the first partner, or simply because they believe the change is not warranted. The dance becomes conflicted and both partners may display anger or frustration.

This dance is interrupted when one partner directly balks at the other's directiveness. It is seen as an order to change, a demand or a threat. In some instances, there is verbal shoving and emotional stepping on the other's feet.

3rd dance pattern: the "Separate" dance
Positive
This dance allows for each partner to be themselves. Both are comfortable and secure in focusing their interests away from each other and on to different activities, things or people. The relationship is maintained but partners may experience certain things apart from one another; this reflects a degree of trust in one another. In this dance, we allow for differences. We feel good about our relationship and even our time apart is wonderful since we know that when we come together, we will share and celebrate each other.

Negative
In this pattern of separate dance, both partners spend all their energy on outside activities. They are not psychologically present for one another; this state could be due to inability or to unwillingness to be in tune with one another. They are, in fact, two ships passing in the night.

EXERCISE

Think back to the video *Husbands and Wives* and try to determine which type of interpersonal dance the couples were doing.

GABE and JUDY

JACK and SALLY

What about ME and YOU?

Recommended Resources

1. Ables, Billie S. *For Couples Only*
   Humanics New Age, Georgia, 1987
2. Beattie, Melody. *Codependent No More*
   Harper/Hazelden Books, San Francisco, 1987
3. Coché, Judith and Erich Coché. *Couples Groups*
   Brunner/Mazel Publishers, New York, 1990
4. Halpern, Howard. *How to Break Your Addiction to a Person*
   Bantam Books, New York, 1982
5. Kiersey, D. and Marilyn Bates. *Please Understand Me*
   Prometheus Nemesis Company, Del Mar, CA, 1984
6. McKay, M., M. Davis, and P. Fanning. *Messages*
   New Harbinger Publications, 1983
7. Miller, Sherod, Daniel Wackman, Elam Nunally, and Phyllis Miller. *Connecting*
   Interpersonal Communication Programs, Inc., CO, 1988
8. ———. *Talking and Listening Together*
   Interpersonal Communication Programs, Inc., CO, 1991
9. Sellner, Judith and James Sellner. *Between the Sexes*
   Self-Counsel Series, Toronto, 1986
10. Westheimer, Ruth. *Dr. Ruth's Guide for Married Lovers*
    Wings Books, New York, 1986
11. Young-Eisendrath, Polly. *Hags and Heroes*
    Inner City Books, Toronto, 1984

CHAPTER 7

CAREER

"Who am I? Am I who I am, or am I what I do?"
– L. Giroux

In this chapter the focus will be on career, that is, what I do as a person, my work. The meaning of "career" as I see it, includes managing a home, going out every morning to a work place, as well as retirement. It encompasses more than the job for which I am remunerated. Some people have a variety of careers simultaneously during their lifetime. For the sake of simplicity, I will maintain that your career is the task-oriented part of your life at present.

Have you ever listed priorities for yourself, and if so, where do you place your career in this priorities list? If you were given an award of excellence in your job, what was it for? Which type of leadership style do you utilize in working with others? If you imagine your own retirement party, what sorts of things might people want to say of you? These are some of the ideas that we will toss around in this chapter on career.

Case Study

Gert, a teacher, is a middle-aged woman, stylish and professional looking. After a few moments of small talk, it becomes obvious that she is in a grave state of depression. She reports sleeping all day long, or wanting to do so. She isolates herself from any social activity and becomes very warm whenever she even thinks of going back into the classroom. It has been two months since Gert has worked. She adds that her physician does not recommend that she return to work yet.

In retrospect, Gert reports how her parents were extremely proud of her choice of teaching as a career; her father always introduced her as "my daughter the teacher." With the therapist, she examines how her career has become her identity. Although she is a mother, a wife, a house manager, a volunteer at the hospital, a coach for a little league baseball team and a reader at Sunday Mass, Gert views herself as a teacher. Now that she cannot perform in this capacity, for whatever reasons, she has lost her sense of dignity and worse than that, her sense of self.

When the therapist suggests that she draw up a list of priorities in her life, it becomes apparent that her energies, both emotional and physical have been almost entirely tied up in her teaching career. There has been little left for her partner and lately for her son; of course, she herself, is at the end of the list. This makes the diagnosis of depression so obvious.

Somehow Gert has become caught in the competition trap, taking summer courses year after year, so as not to appear less qualified than her colleagues. Even her wardrobe is a competitive statement, since she spends unbelievable amounts of money on the newest fashions, in order to keep up with her peers.

The treatment involved going back to the core self-esteem realm, that inside map and chart of what makes Gert a special person with her own uniqueness, regardless of her job. It took some time for her to define herself according to her value system, her personal journey and personal achievements. Also, she needed to eradicate the parental messages that played in her head about "the daughter the teacher." Many exercises in building core self-esteem were introduced and very gradually her identity as a person began to emerge, an identity not directly related to her career.

In due time, she realized that she had a choice in her career situation and she chose to terminate her teaching and to study accounting. Why not? Gert learned that she had many choices that she could make freely and test out the results. No one was allowed to take away that decision-making process from her. As a result, her family saw major changes in her personality and in her moods. Prior to this awareness she had been depressed and angry most of the time, now she had a bounce in her step and was clearly happier with herself than ever before.

EXERCISE IN SONG

The chosen selection is *Old and Wise* from Alan Parsons Project. This song is particularly appropriate for reflection on one's achievements, or career. Envision yourself having reached your 80s or 90s as you listen to this song.

This is a writing exercise for a newspaper. Imagine celebrating your 100th birthday in your local community. Write a short article to accompany your photograph in the newspaper.

Exercise in Film

The film is *Baby Boom,* starring Diane Keaton. Like so many thousands of women in the '80s, the leading lady finds herself juggling her career outside her home with her career inside her home and, more precisely, her identity pre-motherhood and post-motherhood. You may wish to read the writing exercise before you view the film, as a way of focusing your attention.

1. Casey, as we meet her at the beginning of the movie, talks of nothing other than her career. How do you view this one dimensional sort of mind set?

2. She says, "I like work." Does she really like it or is her relationship to it better described in another way?

3. What is your response to the senior partner's statement, "Do you realize the sacrifices you'll have to make if you become a partner in our firm?"

4. What sorts of changes in her lifestyle does Casey need to make with the arrival of the baby?

5. How do the people in Casey's life react to her becoming a mother?

6. As you view this story, does any of it speak to you in terms of some of the challenges you have undergone or anticipate meeting?

WORKAHOLISM

More and more we know that work-related stress is a major cause of concern for all of us at some point in our lives. The following exercises touch a variety of areas where you may want to raise your awareness or make necessary changes. If you choose to go through these exercises by yourself, feel free to give yourself permission to consult with a confidant or a professional should the need arise, depending on the awareness you reach and the sorts of changes you may choose to make.

ALCOHOL + ADDICTION = ALCOHOLISM
SEX + ADDICTION = SEXAHOLISM
DRUGS + ADDICTION = DRUGAHOLISM
SOMETHING + ADDICTION = SOMETHINGAHOLISM
therefore
WORK + ADDICTION = WORKAHOLISM

EXERCISE

Answer yes or no, to the best of your ability.

1. Has anyone in your family or any of your friends ever brought up the subject of your working too hard or constantly?

2. Does your work take up almost all of your time, so that there is none left for your spouse?

3. Have you often needed to cancel going to your children's sports or other activities because of work?

4. Do you carry a cassette recorder so that you can record ideas related to work?

5. Do you draw up a to-do list daily at your job?

6. If something needs to be done around the house, can you sit and relax, and then do the work once you've rested, or is it a *must* to attack the chore immediately?

7. Have you ever had ulcers or other digestive problems after you have had lunch at work?

8. Do you have difficulty delegating to others?

9. Do you often think that you do a better and a quicker job than others, so you tend to do things yourself?

10. Do you find yourself canceling dentist or doctor's appointments because work is too hectic?

11. Do you prefer a social activity directly related to work?

12. Is your work a large part of your conversation?

13. How about vacations? Would you take work-related files and catch up on things?

14. Do you sleep well or do you toss and turn when a work-related situation bothers you?

15. When you introduce yourself, do you say what your job is?

16. Do you fear retirement?

17. Are there any other people in your family of origin who are/were compulsive and addictive?

18. Are you easily obsessed with ideas, people or things?

19. Did you ever have difficulty breaking a bad habit? Smoking, drinking too much caffeine, etc...

20. Do you spend less than 2 half days a week in relaxation, or with your favorite hobby?

All "Yes" answers are indicative of workaholic patterns.

After having read through these questions, my sense is that I have...
a) absolutely none
b) very few
c) some
d) a few
e) many
f) a great many
    ...characteristics of workaholism.

Here is what I intend to do about these traits in my character and behavior:
a) keep myself in check on a daily basis
b) ask a good friend to let me know if I am overdoing things
c) check my overall health

d) or _____

    and _____

    as well as _____

SELF-ESTEEM

Who would ever expect that a famous international movie star has low self-esteem? If you glance through many biographies of the great stars, you will find a considerable number. How can this be? Although the stage lights and the millions of adoring fans yell out "YOU'RE GREAT!" that message does not register deep into the core of the person. Worse yet, it leaves them as before, feeling low in self-esteem. No matter the quality and the quantity of the outside messages, if one does not view the core of their self-worth in a positive way, their self-esteem will be mostly low. It must be an "inside job."

In an outstanding best seller, *Revolution from Within* (Toronto: Little, Brown and Company Ltd., p. 66), Gloria Steinem distinguishes between these two types of self-esteem; she labels them "situational" and "core":

> "This conviction of being loved and lovable, valued and valuable as we are, regardless of what we do, is the beginning of the most fundamental kind of self-esteem: what psychologists call "global" or "characterological" or (the term I find most descriptive because it connotes something that comes first) "core" self-esteem...

> "Later in childhood, we begin to develop the second and more externalized kind of self-esteem, which psychologists call "situational" – the sort that comes from knowing we are good "at" something, compare well with others, meet other people's expectations, and can complete ever more challenging and interesting tasks for the sheer joy of it...

> "The needy child of the past is a kind of emotional black hole into which external rewards disappear..."

Once we become aware of the quality of our self-esteem, which is the source of our emotional life, we can gain important knowledge into how we in fact experience our life. This new-found knowledge provides no immediate and, even sometimes, no possible remedy. However, the sheer awareness of our self-esteem and taking an intense look at where it stems from, prove to be very effective in everyone's unique journey into personhood. A whole and integrated person has developed sufficient core self-esteem to weather the storms that life's roll of the dice brings or the wrong decisions that one makes along the road. A person lacking in core self-esteem and operating on situational factors for self-definition will most often experience a great deal of negative qualifying of who they are.

PRESCRIPTION: TAKING STOCK

I feel good about "me" when...

1.

2.

3.

4.

5.

6.

7.

8.

9.

10.

Once you have listed your stock, you might want to determine whether the self-esteem incidents you have listed are related to "core" or to "situation." After having done this, you will gain a better perspective of your major source of self-esteem boosts. The idea is to draw upon the situational, and to use its positive input as a source of self-confidence. More importantly, however, the intent is to begin transferring the situational instances to core instances, whereby you can be your own best fan. It all boils down to this: if we are not our best admirer, no amount of admiration from the external world will fill the void and give us contentment in the self-esteem arena.

Prescription: Happy Retirement

Time has a way of creeping up on us, and so we commonly hear people express their surprise and amazement that already it is time to retire from a job. We also notice that, in recent years, the age of retirement is considerably younger than it was in the past. Many people have a fulfilling and productive second half of their lives after their first-career years.

Exercise

Imagine that you are asked to assist a cherished colleague in preparing the speech at your retirement party. What would you like this person to say about your working career?

Dear Colleagues and Friends,

Happy Retirement to

RECOMMENDED RESOURCES

1. Greenwald, Jerry. *Be the Person You Were Meant to Be*
   Dell Publishing Co., New York, NY, 1973
2. Hanson, Peter. *The Joy of Stress*
   Collins Publishers, Toronto, 1989
3. ———. *Stress for Success*
   Collins Publishers, Toronto, 1990
4. Hodgson, Ray and Peter Miller. *Self-Watching*
   Methuen Publications, Agincourt, ON, 1982
5. Peale, Norman Vincent. *You Can if You Think You Can*
   Fawcett Crest Books, 1974
6. Powell, John. *Why Am I Afraid to Tell You Who I Am?*
   Argus Communications, Texas, 1969
7. Robertiello, Richard. *Your Own True Love*
   Richard Marek Publishers, New York, 1978
8. Steinem, Gloria. *Revolution from Within*
   Little, Brown and Company Ltd., Toronto, 1992, 1993
9. Twerski, Abraham. *Like Yourself*
   Prentice Hall Press, Toronto, 1978

CHAPTER 8

PARENTING

"Parenting: Did I apply for this job? Do I still want it?"
– L. Giroux

For this noble and unique profession, I was not trained, I was not licensed, and I was not prepared. Much of how I parent is by trial and error, based on my recollection of how I was parented, with a blend of the advice from other parents and from the experts. Parenting is the challenge of one's life I believe. Not only has this been my personal experience but also this has been how parenting is spoken of by my many clients, my colleagues, my family and friends. Most parents do the best that they can and must be commended for their efforts. Without specific instruction being available, such as "Parenting 101," we have discovered that positive validation and encouragement of positive self-esteem are two of the most powerful tools we have to effectively parent. These seem to influence the outcome more than other techniques.

Have you tried to parent your child through contract setting? Does your child experience being appreciated by his or her parents? Is there any verbal or tangible expression of this appreciation? Does your family system have a hierarchy? What role does your child play in making decisions concerning the parenting itself? These are some of the controversial issues that we will discuss in this chapter.

CASE STUDY

As the Smith family enter the therapist's office, they take various chairs while the therapist observes where each member chooses to sit. The position where each member selects to sit can be of significance to the dynamic of this family system. Mother has set up the appointment, reporting that there is major upheaval at home; she adds that Samantha is the problem. Father accompanies the family this morning, making certain that everyone is aware that he has taken off from work to be here. Bobby moves a chair as far away from the family circle as he possibly can and slouches as only a teenaged boy with long lanky legs can. Tim moves in very close to his mom and complains immediately about his allergic reaction to "something" in this office. As for Samantha, she is clutching her doll with whom she is having conversation.

Whenever the therapist asks a question of anyone in the family system, Mother immediately answers, in effect being the spokesperson for the family. She appears intent on explaining how Samantha is the problem since she is spoiled by her father and older brothers. This little seven-year-old refuses to go to bed at night and throws tantrums when she is disciplined. In the past, she has bitten her mother. Her treatment of her siblings is somewhat better than her treatment of her parents. Samantha, herself, reports that she hates her mother because she is too bossy.

Bobby sits away from the system and rocks back and forth on the chair. He wears a cap which conceals his eyes and one wonders if he can see anything at all. Quickly he responds to the therapist, when addressed, that he does not want to be here; Mom is the one with the problem and Dad is out of it completely. Bobby adds that his mom watches too many talk shows and has become lost in the "go to the therapist" scene. When asked how he gets along with Samantha, Bobby reports that she is fine as long as you let her do what she wants.

During the session so far, Tim has blown his nose very loudly and is so close to his mother that one would think he is sitting on her lap. He has nothing to report or to add to what Bobby has said. "I don't know..." is his only response. At one point, he whispers in Mother's ear, "Can we go now?" At this, his mother replies that once the session is over, she will take him for a nice cold drink and perhaps ice cream also. She tells him that all this commotion has upset him and that is why his allergies are acting up. Mother reports that Tim has nothing to do with his sister at all, that Samantha usually shouts that he is a crybaby and prefers to have nothing to do with him either.

Father sighs repeatedly during the session and says very little. When Samantha makes her remarks, her dad gives her a stern look but says nothing. When the therapist asks Father a direct question, he steers to Mother so that she will answer for him. A few times, Father asks Bobby to sit up straight and Tim to stop blowing his nose so loud. Before the session is over, Father says he must leave and return to the office, that Mother can handle things very well. As he leaves, Bobby's look is resentful and Samantha teases Tim with the box of Kleenex.

The therapist stops the session at this point and requests to see the parents without the children for the next session. The work will involve strengthening the couple system, the executive of the family, before the children can be brought in for sessions. It is quite obvious that Bobby is angry with his dad, that Mother is taking way too much control in this system, that Tim needs to individuate from his mother, and that Samantha is playing on everyone's weaknesses. The prognosis depends on how well the couple can effectively communicate, followed with some action plan to enhance the family cohesiveness. Boundaries will need to be set between individual members as well as between the parents and the children.

EXERCISE IN SONG

The chosen selection is the popular song *The Greatest Love*, by Whitney Huston. It suggests that the most precious gift we can give our children is love of self. Listen to it and record for yourself the awareness it raises around the issue of parenting.

1. How do I encourage my child to develop his/her self-esteem?

2. Who are my child's heroes?

3. Am I an effective parent?

4. What does my child think of me as a parent?

5. Does my own level of self-esteem contribute to my child's self-esteem?

Exercise in Film

Although the film *Parenthood*, starring Steve Martin, is classified as a comedy, it explores various methods of parenting and presents a serious look at four family systems. We meet parents in a traditional family using a commonsense approach, two families with single parents, one struggling to control her kids and the other treating his son as a "buddy," and finally parents representing the scholarly approach that focuses on giving the child a vast variety of knowledge. Watch the video and then do the following writing exercise.

Four Family Systems

The following are four skeleton genograms, each one representing one of the families in the film.

#1

■ ● Gil and Karen (dad and mom)

■ Kevin

● Taylor

■ Justin

#2
● Helen (mom)
● Julie
■ Gary

#3
■ ● Nathan and Susan (dad and mom)
● Patti

#4
■ Larry (dad)
■ Cool

Food for thought

For each of these family systems, think about the following:

1. Which type of parenting goes on? What characterizes it?

2. What quality of life do the children have?

3. What is the possible outcome of the parenting in this system?

4. Can I relate to any of these systems? How?

PRESCRIPTION: CONTRACTING

The term "contracting" is used to designate a technique in which we promote responsibility and communication with another person. The process involves talking about and listening to an issue, followed by a direct involvement on the part of the person who is willing to change something or to take action on something. In this way, a child or a parent can take responsibility or action at a preset time, a contracted time.

Example

During a session, Susan shares with her therapist that she is experiencing a profound need to have a heart-to-heart talk with her mother, with whom she has had a falling out. After some deliberation, Susan reports being seriously committed to calling her mother; this is when the therapist suggests contracting this issue.

On a blank piece of paper, Susan writes the date and location, followed by a very simple contract such as: "On_____, I,_____will call my mother_____ to initiate a conversation between us." Both Susan and the therapist sign the contract.

It is imperative that the person committing to the contract be willing and ready to do so; usually, pressure does not bring about positive results. Contracting is a graphic expression and an outward representation of a commitment already made to oneself. Contracting may be done on paper or verbally.

Example

Upon arriving at her mother's home for a visit, Susan notices her brother's car in the driveway. Because there is a history of conflict with this sibling, she simply contracts with herself, "During this visit, I will keep cool around my brother and not allow him to push my buttons."

Such a very simple contract raises Susan's level of awareness and provides a sort of game plan for her visit. There is a certain experience of empowerment rendered by the "contracting."

Contracting with my child

- Choose a very simple situation where it is apparent that your child is intent on taking action to change a behavior, thought, or action.
- Invite the child to draw up their own contract with you.
- Both child and adult sign or draw their signature.

Typical issues

- Leaving personal belongings lying around the house.
- Putting dirty dishes into the dishwasher.
- Interrupting people when they are talking.
- Sharing time and toys with siblings.

Certificate of appreciation

One of our basic human needs is validation. Children, even at a very young age, thrive on validation. This exercise presents a technique called "certificate of appreciation." It can be awarded daily, weekly, monthly or at various occasions to validate and positively stroke a child. It does not mean that the child will strive to be perfect, but rather that the child will realize how he or she is appreciated by their mom and dad. Efforts, as well as successes, should be rewarded by appreciation. On the following page is a simple example of a certificate given to a child.

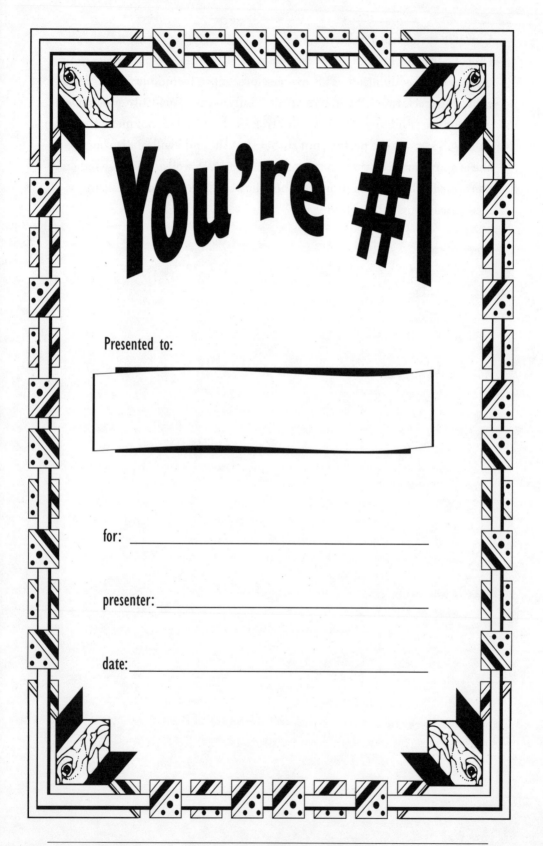

You're #1

Presented to:

for: _____

presenter: _____

date: _____

Prescription: Family Cohesion

A family system's cohesion is the glue that keeps it together. We may refer to it as unity or the feeling of being part of something. There are some basic guidelines that we can follow with our own children in order to promote cohesion in our family system.

Autonomy
While parents work diligently at a close relationship with their children, each child is encouraged to develop their own autonomy.

Action not the child
Parents may be critical towards a behavior but not critical towards the child: "What you have DONE is bad."

Child's opinion
A child may have a different opinion or be different themself and still have a right to parental support.

Only if you're good
The relationship between the parent and the child must be independent of the behavior of the child.

Mistakes
A child is allowed to make mistakes.

Admitting to a mistake
Parents who can admit their mistakes to their children are the best examples for their children to follow.

If family cohesion were a simple task, no one would bother to write about it. There are countless "experts" who will claim the same types of ideals and objectives; those are only the general rules we can try to maintain. We do the best we can with what we have. Attaining a comfortable level of cohesion is the ultimate goal.

PRESCRIPTION: FAMILY MEETINGS

When the Smith family returned home from their first session with the therapist, Mother insisted they have their first family meeting right then and there. Needless to say that Bobby's rude remarks to her, Tim's sniffling and whining, and Samantha's outburst when she discovered one of the plush toys being eaten by the new puppy were not conducive to trying a new technique designed to promote family unity. Probably, the reason why family meetings have gotten a bad reputation in the past is that they have been conducted at the wrong time or in the wrong way.

The secret to effective family meetings: keep them brief and enjoyable.

Only if the experience of the family meeting is a positive one will the members of the family be interested in making it a practice. And only when it becomes a regular practice does it offer the full value of its possibilities.

About the family meeting

Who?   All members of the family.

When?   A time when all members are available. The end of a meal is a common time used.

What?   A time for each individual member to share with others how he or she is experiencing their system. Families can brainstorm a specific topic when it is warranted, e.g., a vacation.

How?   It is imperative that each member have their voice, that one person chair the meeting so as to allow each person to take their turn talking.

Frequency? Every few weeks, with each meeting lasting for only a few minutes until all members have had an opportunity to speak.

Recommendations

- Asking each member of the family system to chair the meeting adds variety and also a sense of validation to smaller children.
- The intent is not to solve all the problematic situations but merely to discuss openly and to give each member a chance to be heard.
- One way to enhance the family meeting is by also making it the "certificate of appreciation" time.

- Post the upcoming family meeting on the calendar or on the refrigerator to allow members to think about what they would like to bring up at the meeting.
- Encourage positive feedback when sharing during the meeting; in some systems, members must balance every negative comment with a positive one.

PLAN OF ACTION

THE _____ FAMILY MEETING

TO BE HELD ON _____

AT _____

TOPICS OF DISCUSSION _____

_____

_____

CHAIRPERSON _____

ATTENDANCE **COMPULSORY**

Recommended Resources

1. Beavers, Robert and Robert Hampson. *Successful Families*
   W.W. Norton & Company, New York, 1990
2. Dinkmeyer, Don & Gary McKay. *Step, The Parents' Handbook*
   American Guidance Service, Circle Pines, MN, 1976
3. Efron, Don. *The Strategic Parenting Manual*
   J.S.S.T., London, 1980
4. Faber, Adele and Elaine Mazlish. *Liberated Parents, Liberated Children*
   Avon, Publishers of Bard, Camelot and Discus Books, 1975
5. Greenleaf, Barbara Kaye. *Help: A Handbook for Working Mothers*
   Berkley Publishing Corporation, 1980
6. Hoffman, Lynn. *Foundations of Family Therapy*
   Basic Books Inc., Publishers, New York
7. Levine, Saul. *Tell Me It's Only A Phase*
   Prentice-Hall Canada Inc., Scarborough, ON, 1987
8. Miller, Sherod. *Connecting with Self and Others*
   Interpersonal Communications Programs, Inc., Littleton, CO, 1988
9. Peck, Ellen and Dr. William Granzig. *The Parent Test*
   G.P. Putnam's Sons, New York, 1978
10. Self-Counsel, Marion Crook, ed. *Please, Listen to Me!*
    Self-Counsel Press, Canada, 1992
11. York Phyllis. *Toughlove Solutions*
    Bantam Books, Toronto, 1984

CHAPTER 9

TOPSY-TURVY:

ILLNESS

*"The world breaks everyone and afterward many
are strong at the broken places..."*
– Ernest Hemingway

Rather than title this chapter of the workbook, "living with illness," I chose to name it "Topsy-Turvy" since in effect, when one lives with chronic illness, one's life, every area of it, goes into disarray. The experience of living through and within this mode is unique and unless one has actually been immersed in it, one has only an outsider's perspective of it. For the caregiver, there is also much change and adaptation. This chapter is dedicated to and focuses on chronic illness from the eyes of a chronically ill person; therefore, the exercises will be geared as such. A great number of caregivers and people associated with them might benefit from going through the exercises with a challenged person.

Some of the questions we will be looking at are:
• What is my vision of myself as a chronically ill person?
• How do I process my anger at the fact that life has dealt me this bad hand?
• Can I change my priorities, my behaviors and my thinking to meet the challenge successfully?
• Do I manage my anger or does it manage me?
• Are there any practical activities that can assist in my anger management?
• In terms of stages of grieving my losses, where am I presently?
• Do I encourage wellness or illness in my life?
• What are positive ways of grieving the losses brought on by illness?

CASE STUDY

When Leah enters her therapist's office for her first session, she quickly reports that her family has suggested that she seek help. The fact that she has recently been diagnosed with multiple sclerosis has not altered her life as far as she is concerned; she reports how she is just "fine" and coping well. It is only when the therapist begins to probe into her "feelings" that there is an apparent freeze in this area. The client is in shock and feels numb, which is not uncommon to newly diagnosed people.

On the second visit, Leah begins to open up about how this news has affected her husband, Bob. Apparently, he has shut down his affections and his communication. When she needs to see her physician, Bob has an excuse for not being available to accompany her. Leah has heard and has read about the statistics concerning marriage breakdown after diagnosis of chronic illness, and she fears that the end of her relationship is near. Her partner is not able to cope with how this disease affects her life and with the other losses that it might bring.

For the last 15 years, Leah held an executive position with a bank; at present, she is on a long-term disability plan because she cannot work. Her exhaustion is acute and she needs to nap several times during the day. With the loss of her identity as a career woman, Leah has lost a great deal of self-esteem and self-confidence. She is 35 years old and already into the world of retirement. Much of her day is spent lying around in her nightgown, watching television and self-destructing with cigarettes, alcohol and over-the-counter sleeping aids. She sees herself as a "has-been," her body has let her down and she has joined the club of the walking dead.

When Leah was productive and not physically challenged, she had a reputation for her fashion style. These days, there is no make-up or doing her hair or dressing up; her sexuality is totally dormant and her sexual desires are nil. When she thinks about her past sex life, Leah experiences a part of her that she believes to be dead and numbed, like her genitalia is, because of the multiple sclerosis. She reports that she cannot wear skirts because the only shoes she can walk in are flat; she has given her high-heeled shoes to a charity. Bob has not touched her in months now, and that is exactly what she prefers.

To her surprise and amazement, her teenaged son has been getting into trouble at school. He has become somewhat obnoxious, a different boy than previously. Leah finds a poem he has written about illness, in which she reads of his sorrow regarding his mother's illness, yet he never verbalizes what is going on inside of him. When she tries to reprimand him, the boy retorts that she is too weak to discipline him anymore and does not take her seriously.

The home that Bob and Leah had built was inappropriate to meet her needs. They would need to find another place where Leah could have everything within the house accessible to her. Bob is disheartened because he spent so much time and energy on their first home, their son does not want to leave his friends and his school, and Leah sees herself as the awful culprit who caused all of this upheaval. At this time she feels much guilt and disgust for what she has become, and admits that the illness has won over her.

Many of her friends have not contacted her for several months; perhaps they think she is contagious!!! Leah is well aware of their awkwardness and inability to cope. "What do I say" and "what do I do," they wonder. Even if she realizes that this is a normal reaction, she still misses the interaction and the socializing. With her family of origin, it's been much the same. Some of her siblings are into guilt because she became afflicted and they didn't, some are in denial of the whole thing and pretend it is not happening, and some still hurt too much to get close to her or to invite her to disclose what she is experiencing.

The therapy involves grief work concerning all the losses that Leah has experienced. Defining herself all over again, finding a blend of her old identity and her new identity will be the next step. Gradually, Leah will find her own power and strength to manage, to cope, and to face her challenges; she will draw on determination she never knew she had. Along the way, she finds a network of people with whom she increases her positive coping skills and shares her enthusiasm to win the war against her disease. Leah will learn not to apologize because she is physically challenged; to ask for her needs to be met in accordance with the chronic illness; and she will find another peace, another way out.

EXERCISE IN SONG

The song selection for this chapter on illness and its challenges is *Man in Motion* (theme song from *St. Elmo's Fire*). It was Rick Hansen's theme song as he propelled his wheelchair across the highways of Canada, inspiring and empowering thousands of challenged people to courage and to hope. The chosen song is a good place to begin to develop your awareness of how you are meeting the challenge of illness.

You may want to listen to the song a few times. As you do so, pick out three phrases, expressions or words that speak very clearly to you; they will most likely be areas where you can identify with the "man in motion." Allow yourself to write freely about how these words speak particularly to you. If you find yourself getting into feelings, that is a positive sign that you are becoming aware of your experience with illness.

1. Phrase from song

   How does it speak to you?

2. Phrase from song

   How does it speak to you?

3. Phrase from song

   How does it speak to you?

EXERCISE IN FILM

The film selection is *Passion Fish*. Before you view the film and do the exercise to accompany it, read through the following brief explanation on the stages of grieving as they apply to chronic illness. Following the notes on the grieving process, the exercise to accompany the film will be presented.

STAGES OF GRIEVING
ILLNESS = LOSSES = GRIEVING

1. I can't believe IT... I am frozen in shock.	SHOCK
2. I won't believe IT... I am numb with sadness.	DEPRESSION
3. I am ready to look at IT... I am angry or depressed.	ANGER
4. I am moving towards IT... I am frightened.	FEAR
5. I dance with IT... I am recycled.	ACCEPTANCE

Shock
At this first stage of grieving, one is in a state of shock. Usually feelings are frozen: a safety device. The person cannot allow him or herself to believe that they are afflicted; "this can't be happening to me..." The fact that illness has hit so close to home is unbelievable, and if the person doesn't allow themself to believe it then they think they don't need to deal with it. At this stage one goes on with his or her life, sometimes as if nothing has occurred. There is a great deal of denial at this stage of grieving.

Depression
At some point, the person begins to consider the possibility of illness having actually stricken them. Usually the smallest indication of being able

to believe it brings, along with this awareness, a refusal to believe. In order to maintain this level of non-belief, one isolates; other people in their life may support the truth and the "patient" refuses to handle this truth. A level of depression develops from the isolation.

Anger

The depression begins to lift when the patient begins to process their anger. There is valid reason to be angry: this is not fair! At this stage, the person will search out a target to blame or to rage at; this can be very healthy and, more than that, quite necessary to achieve effective grieving. Things to consider are effective anger processing techniques – those which do not harm anyone, neither the patient nor people in their life. If the patient begins to turn the rage inward, this can result in suicide – the ultimate self-destructive route. Therefore it is imperative to seek help and assistance in order to live through the anger and the rage in an appropriate way. If the anger reaches raging proportions, it can be monitored to assure that it is healthily and effectively processed.

Fear

By this time, the person has much awareness of their own illness and diseased condition. Now the fear sets in. The fear of dying painfully, the fear of one's caregivers hurting from compassion, the fear of pain, the fear of the slow corrosion of one's health, the fear of being labeled, the fear of unemployment, the fear of poverty, the fear of losing one's partner: all of these represent major fears experienced by the chronically ill person. Allowing oneself to express the fear diminishes its impact. There is no fear greater than the fear faced in isolation. After all, fear is often "False Evidence Appearing Real." If the fear is based on reality, one will develop the coping mechanism necessary at the appropriate time.

Acceptance

In contrast with the "peaceful waters" imagery that the term acceptance conjures up, acceptance is born of the actual tempestuous sea where one has to sail before they get to the calm waters. It is a place one comes to after a long climb through numbed feelings, tears and fears. A sense of peace accompanies this stage of grieving; there seems to be a quiet mode of "just going on with life" minus the losses. People display creativity at this stage

– innovative ways of coping with a healthy degree of contentment with one's life as it is. It is in effect dancing with the illness.

Note: It is common for a person to experience various stages of grieving more than once. For example, any remission in the illness will produce denial and a false sense of new truth. Of course, when the illness takes its course once again, the patient goes back to step 1. In most cases, the second, third or any subsequent slip into "depression," for example, will not be as lengthy nor as profoundly draining as the initial experience of the stage of depression. Especially when a patient has the knowledge that the painful stage has ended before, there is hope that it will do so once more.

EXERCISE

Having viewed the film *Passion Fish*, try to determine how the challenged woman experiences the various stages of grieving the loss of her physical wholeness. You can do this by filling in the following blanks:

1. When she...

   ...she is experiencing SHOCK.

2. We notice the following signs of her DEPRESSION...

3. She expresses her ANGER by...

4. When she ...

... she is in her ANGER stage.

5. At the point when she...

... we recognize that she is in the ACCEPTANCE stage.

6. My pattern of grieving.

I am in shock when...

I am in depression when...

I am in anger when...

I am in fear when...

I am in acceptance when...

PRESCRIPTION:
I'M SO ANGRY I COULD...

Anger is... is not...

ANGER is an emotional reaction to a primary emotion.

ANGER is a way in which one copes with that primary emotion.

ANGER is a defense against pain or fear.

ANGER is not a positive or a negative emotion, but rather just an emotion.

ANGER can range from mild irritation to full blown rage, as in suicide.

ANGER is not always focused outward.

ANGER can be masked in depression, sarcasm or humor.

ANGER, when repressed, can create physiological conditions such as heart disease.

ANGER has potential to isolate the person who is stuck in it.

Anger and Illness

ANGER is created by a sense of loss of control and chronic illness is all about loss of control.

ANGER is a protection against sadness and pain caused by illness.

ANGER comes in waves, as in the stages of grieving.

ANGER is a cry for empathy and support.

ANGER is one of the first reactions to loss.

ANGER looks for a target.

ANGER is more intense because of the "no win" situation of chronic illness.

My Anger Triggers

ANGER is triggered as my list of losses grows longer.

ANGER is triggered as the feeling of abandonment and neglect comes from the family or other caregivers.

ANGER is triggered by certain events: anniversary of last work day, of wedding, of the day of the diagnosis.

ANGER is triggered by comparing myself to others not so incapacitated.

ANGER is triggered by the raised awareness of loss of financial security.

ANGER is triggered by my changed role in the family or the social circuit.

ANGER is triggered while I watch television, listen to the radio, receive a phone call or read a newspaper.

ANGER is triggered by experiencing a violation of my boundaries.

ANGER is triggered by the "well" society's lack of compassion and sensitivity.

I Am Responsible

I am responsible for how I manage my anger.

Illness does not give me a license to become a raging aggressor.

I am accountable for my anger, just as I attempt to maintain my choices.

I am responsible to acknowledge the anger that I feel, that I see, that I hear.

My responsibility (as an attendant) is to listen, to be with the person while they experience their anger.

I am not responsible to fix it (as a caregiver), to change it, to suppress it.

I am responsible for my self-care, both as the one in anger and the one attending.

No No's

- *If I attack* my family, my friends or a medical staff, either physically, verbally or emotionally, I am acting inappropriately.
- *If I repress* by denying, I can become severely depressed and lethargic.
- *I harm myself* by neglecting my condition, by not taking proper medication or by taxing my body too much.
- *I prolong my suffering* if I do not own the primary feelings such as sadness and fear, so I need to investigate beyond the anger.

10+ Management

- *I seek* professional therapy if I feel stuck in the anger.
- *I give* careful consideration to whom I ask to attend to my anger.
- *I verbalize* my anger with raging words if necessary.
- *I draw* a picture of my target and let the picture have the anger.
- *I pound* a pillow or other safe surface.
- *I write* an angry letter and tear it up afterwards, or process it with someone.
- *I give* myself permission to cry for the losses I have.
- *I protect myself* from hooking into others' anger. I do not fight other people's battles.
- *I set limits* to the amount of time for venting anger.
- *I use the anger* as energy to fight for social justice such as the rights of the physically challenged.
- *I use my anger* as energy to maintain my dignity of living.

CONTRACT

RE: ANGER

DATE _____

PLACE _____

I, _____, choose to contract with

you, _____, an agreement in which I

will attempt to effectively manage my anger.

These are some of the changes I am willing to make:

Signatures:

_____

anger manager

_____

attendant

Meeting the challenges

The occurrence of chronic illness brings to the family system many challenges. With these challenges, comes a time of questioning. The following are some of the areas affected and questioned.

The Questions

1. GRIEVING: I am angry or depressed all the time. Will this grieving of my health ever end?

2. CAREGIVER: Although my husband/wife has vowed "in sickness and in health," will s/he be able to handle this?

3. CAREER: Since I don't "do" anymore, who have I become?

4. FINANCES: How will we manage on half of our usual income?

5. SEXUALITY: i) How can I feel like a woman, when I don't have the energy to dress or to make up my face? ii) I've gained so much weight from sitting in my wheelchair. How could any woman find me attractive?

6. SEX: I am always exhausted and sex is the last thing on my mind. Will my partner be able to handle this?

7. PARENTING: How can I be a parent to my children when I have trouble standing up?

8. HOUSING: More and more I cannot climb the stairs nor am I safe in the shower or getting in and out of the bathtub. How could we go about making our home more accessible?

9. FRIENDS: Since I am home from the hospital, my friends seem to have abandoned me. Do they think I have a contagious illness?

10. FAMILY: Nearly every member of my extended family has some miraculous drug or treatment for me to try; they have all become experts. How do I tell them to let me make my choices and still maintain their affections?

My Answers

After taking time to think about the questions arising from the challenges of chronic illness, develop some of your own answers as means of coping and meeting those challenges.

1. My grieving...

2. My caregiver...

3. My job...

4. My finances...

5. My sexuality...

6. My sex life...

7. My parenting...

8. My home...

9. My friends...

10. My family...

Poetry for Wellness

With the ravages of illness, people often experience the loss of certain bodily functions or of certain body parts or organs.

At the time when MS attacked Leah's vision, she came to realize the preciousness of her sight. At first, she anguished through bouts of anger. Because this was not productive, she searched for other methods of coping with her grief. She discovered that a positive and a grateful relationship with her eyes was the key to effective grieving. Following is a poem she wrote to her eyes.

To My Eyes

You gift me with sight

of mountains and lakes and snow

of my son's smile

and

of my lover's smirk.

You open up my universe

in the early morning sunshine.

You bring into my home,

artists, actors, musicians.

With you I travel independently

on country roads, and superhighways,

take my son to a baseball game

and

my lover out for dinner.

But of all the gifts you bestow,

You, my eyes, are the key to seeing into another's soul

and if ever I should lose you

that is what I will grieve the most.

Since poetry is an artful expression of feelings, I recommend poetic verse as an effective vehicle to express one's feelings.

Exercise

This is a writing exercise. Write a poem dedicated to part of your body that is afflicted or has been lost to illness.

My Poem

VISUALIZATION

More than ever before, we are aware of the power of our mind. Our thoughts, our perceptions, our beliefs and our attitude play a major role in living with illness.

The following is an exercise in visualization. It is a tool that you can use in the effective management of your disease and of its symptoms.

Note: Because this sort of exercise can be emotionally draining, I suggest you partake in it with a confidant or a trained professional, to have someone with whom you can do your processing afterward.

In a quiet and safe place, begin a relaxation time. Take deep breaths to the count of 10 and exhale slowly to the count of 10. Repeat this a few times until you are relaxed and comfortable.

In your mind's eye, picture some image that represents your illness.
Is IT a human shape, animal shape, or a natural shape?
Is IT a mineral shape, vegetable, or other form?
What color is IT?
How big is IT?
Where is IT?
How does IT communicate with you?
Observe IT for a moment.
When you are ready, approach IT.
Now speak to IT.
Give IT a name.
What do you need to say to IT?

Processing the experience
How was this visualization experience for you?

What have you learned from it?

Are there any changes that you could bring to your life in coping with your illness?

REMEMBER: "Nothing is impossible... it's just that I haven't done it yet."
— Japanese Proverb

PRESCRIPTION: MEDITATION

The following meditation was created by and for someone whose limbs are affected by multiple sclerosis. She uses soothing instrumental music as a background and a comfortable chair or bed to lie in during her meditation. To create her setting, she has utilized a place where she has experienced peace and love; this engages much of her sensory self in the mind's meditation exercise.

This sort of "wellness" meditation can be adapted easily to suit your own personal situation. An effective way to use it is by recording your own voice as you read through the meditation; this allows for added relaxation when you listen to your meditation as well as an increased sense of personal ownership.

My eyes see the white sandy Caribbean beach of St. John...no one on the beach...all is serene...the palm trees sway back and forth, rocking me in a slumber...the water a perfect blanket of turquoise...so clear that I can see the coral with my naked eye...I hear the gentle strength of the roar of the waves, they sound like praying nuns, chanting a very low, healing chant...

my husband is in the water with his friend... I hear their laughter...my lover/husband is so beautiful... I am filled with awe...I am sitting on the sand, my legs in the water...the waves come to me and soothe my feet...they gently wash and cleanse me of the heat...they lay me down to rest for a minute while they go back for more fresh water...they are caring for me...the world is perfect... I am perfectly content...my heart is filled with love...I am well...my hands can dig into the sand and draw little pictures...my eyes see the magnificent beauty of the coconut trees beyond me...I feel loved and cherished... I rise and walk into the water towards my kindred spirit and we embrace...the waves follow me with more fresh water...this is paradise...I am cooled by the water...

I am held in tender arms...I am perfectly well...I am perfectly well...I am perfectly well...

Exercise: Meditation

This is an exercise in meditation. You can write your own meditation. Select an experience that was very calming for you, one when you felt well. The idea is to focus all of your senses, one at a time, on the setting you have chosen. Include smells, sights, touches, movement, sounds, etc. It is important to make many affirmative statements like, "I am content, I am perfectly well..." You are free to stretch your imagination so that affected limbs or lost faculties can be imagined "well" again. If a musical background is pleasurable to you, then by all means use one when you tape your own voice reading the meditation. This exercise is a way of taking care of yourself, not to mention taking an active role in your wellness.

Recommended Resources

1. Cleveland, Martha. *Living Well*
   Harper & Row Publishers, San Francisco, 1989
2. Coffey-Lewis, Lou. *Be Restored to Health*
   Random House of Canada Limited, Toronto, 1984
3. Cousins, Norman. *Head First, the Biology of Hope*
   E. P. Dutton, Toronto, 1989
4. Frankl, Viktor E. *The Doctor and the Soul*
   Vintage Books, New York, 1986
5. Giroux, Louise. *Recycled: A Story of Hope*
   Fenix Ryzing Associates, Sudbury, Ontario, 1995
6. Hay, Louise. *The Power Is within You*
   Hay House, CA, 1991
7. ———. *You Can Heal Your Life*
   Hay House, CA, 1984
8. LeMaistre, JoAnn. *Beyond Rage*
   Alpine Guild, Illinois, 1985
9. McKay, Rogers & McKay. *When Anger Hurts*
   New Harbinger Publications, CA, 1989
10. Siegel, Bernie. *How to Live between Office Visits*
    Harper Collins Publishers, 1993
11. ———. *Love, Medicine and Miracles*
    Harper and Row Publishers, NY, 1986
12. ———. *Peace, Love and Healing*
    Harper and Row Publishers, NY, 1990
13. Stearns, Ann Kaiser. *Living through Personal Crisis*
    Ballantine Books, NY, 1984

CHAPTER 10

ME & YOU
YOU & ME

"True intimacy with another human being can only be experienced when you have found true peace within yourself."
– A.L. Wozniak

"Me & You, You & Me" focuses on healthy coupleship. How to build a healthy intimate relationship and how to best sustain it is the focus of this chapter. This chapter is intended to supplement chapter six – Couple Relationships.

In these times, couples face many challenges; we are in great need of simple tools that can be utilized to heal or to enhance our relationships. It is my hope that some of these exercises, reflections and ideas will be of benefit to you.

CASE STUDY

After 28 years of married life, Olga and Bert made their first appointment for marriage counseling. They appeared to be in conflict, yet, committed to each other and to their relationship. What the therapist immediately surmised was that they both had very ineffective communication skills. When one spoke, the other did not take time to listen; in fact, neither seemed to know how to listen. They were both quite relieved to learn that communication is much more than speaking or listening; they realized that, for most of their married lives, they had not been connected with each other in an effective, communicative way. The therapist explained how they could learn to communicate effectively if they were willing to learn and if their commitment was strong enough.

Olga and Bert were thrilled at this and actually wanted another session the next day when the therapist scheduled them for the following week. When she assigned the homework to them, they appeared somewhat shocked until the therapist told them about doing the work in a couple system. This was the homework, the questions to be addressed individually and not shared until the next session:

    Do you keep secrets from your spouse?

    What is that all about for you?

    Do you play together as children do?

    What is that all about for you?

    Has your relationship changed over the years? Can you describe how?

    Do you trust your partner when it comes to sharing your feelings?

Do you feel heard when you say something to your partner?

What has kept you together for the past 28 years of your lives?

Olga and Bert were diligent in their homework and the therapy went on for several sessions. The therapist coached them on communication skills and they applied their new-found knowledge in all areas of their lives. It was as though they were courting all over again. Once they became convinced that playing together as children was healthy and necessary to healthy relationship, they let go of their inhibitions. At one session, Olga wore a pendant with a bottle for blowing bubbles and reported that her boyfriend Bert had surprised her with it. He reported finding a new water gun in his pool shed. The couple was now talking and listening to each other as well as playing now and again.

One of the areas where they needed to do some work was in the "phase" dimension of their relationship. (More about phases later in this chapter.) Now that their children had left home, they needed to adapt to this new place. Both reported not knowing what it was all about, but somehow had experienced the last year as very different and empty since the last child left.

At some points in their new way of relating, Olga and Bert discovered things they had never realized about each other. They learned to compromise much more and to not keep anything from each other for very long; the therapist had called this "plaque build-up" that needed to be discarded and talked over as soon as possible.

Bert and Olga joined a communication for couples group for six sessions, under the recommendation of their therapist. There they witnessed that they were not alone; they made contact with other couples who had experienced some of the same areas of difficulty.

It was at the last session of this skills group that Bert called the therapist aside to show her a beautiful wedding band; he was to give it to his bride Olga on their trip to Disney World where they were heading for a vacation of play and intimacy. Bert's eyes shone with love for his Olga and pride in himself for his courage to "do the work."

EXERCISE IN SONG

The song selection, *Storybook Love,* is from the movie *The Princess Bride*. It is a very romantic and traditional love song, the type where the couple ride off into the sunset. Because my intent is to promote a healthy and "happy ever after" style of relationship, the choice was made deliberately to display romance and true love.

It is true that more often than not, your fantasy romance is light years from your real-life relationship. Day-to-day living routines, unexpected events, illness and death, financial stress and many other factors make real life a drama more than a fantasy ride. What I am proposing is a healthy escape into perhaps a prior time when you've experienced the feelings of a fantasy romance or an imagined time when you'll find your partner and you in such a fantasy. I want to focus on the possibilities only, on the beautiful character traits that both of you have; let's neglect all the negative attributes and the habits and the ruts you might have fallen into in your relationship. The exercise is designed to encourage you to make a decision and a genuine attempt at seeing your partner in a "fantastic" light.

As you listen to the selection, enjoy a little fantasy in the marriage-made-in-heaven mode. An exercise to accompany the song will follow.

EXERCISE

Now that you have enjoyed the selection, I invite you to write a short fairy tale, or storybook-love type of story about your own relationship. Perhaps it could be for your children, your grandchildren or the inner child of any adult who wants to read a beautiful love story. The characters will be you and your partner.

Our Storybook Love...

The Author...

EXERCISE IN FILM

The film selection for this chapter is a very beautiful fantasy called *The Princess Bride*. It is indeed a collector's item for your video library and a welcome addition to any home. Your sense of timing in watching this film with your partner is important. Let it be a special time, with popcorn, peace and quiet, pajamas, or whatever else would make it a unique time for the two of you.

This is a note writing exercise. Both you and your partner will write each other a love-note which you will then share. A good time to do this exercise is right after watching the film.

Dear Prince,

all my love,

Dear Princess,

all my love,

EXERCISE:
THE WISH GAME FOR COUPLES

Materials

a blanket and pillows

a loving and willing couple

20 wish cards (prepared earlier by the couple)

a die

candles

2 small bowls

1. Instructions

Prior to the game, each of the partners prepares 10 wish cards for the game. These wish cards are to be suitable for the privacy of your home and with a limited time given to make the wish come true. These wishes may range from, " I wish you would say... to me," to "I wish you would dance with me," to "I wish you would caress me," to "I wish you would give me a body massage" to any sexual wish agreeable to your partner and to your sexual preferences. The wish cards are folded and kept without sharing them before the game.

2. Setting

Prepare the place where you will engage in your wish game. The setting should be comfortable as well as intimate, safe from distractions. I suggest a living room floor, with blankets and pillows and candles.

3. Players

Only two players may participate. I suggest that each one be relaxed either by taking a warm bath or a shower prior to beginning the wish game. Dress is optional. (Really !!!)

4. Let the game begin

Each partner's wish cards are tossed in a bowl. The player who rolls the highest number on the die begins the game by picking one of his or her own wish cards. The wish is fulfilled. The game continues this way; there is no time limit other than the one the partners might agree to. When one partner's wish cards are all fulfilled, the game is technically over.

5. Personalizing the game

Crack open a bottle of your favorite wine. Prepare a snack for each other to have during the game. You may want to continue fulfilling all of your partner's wishes even if you win the game. PLAY, PLAY, PLAY.

Exercise: Together & Separate

Before doing the following exercise, I recommend you look over the "interpersonal dance" patterns that are noted in chapter six of this workbook. The 3rd dance pattern, the "separate" dance, is the dance I will be referring to in this exercise.

A couple in relationship need to develop a togetherness that incorporates separateness. Both of these positions are of equal importance and, when well balanced, they create an awesome dance pattern for a couple. Each partner remains an individual with his or her own life, interests, preferences, friends, hobbies and so on. At the same time, the couple join together in some activities, interests, with friends, in travel and so on, as one and the same unit. If a person is solely separate, there is no possibility for togetherness. On the other hand, if a couple is always in togetherness, there is no possibility for separateness and one of them is apt to experience codependency. It is a tall order to create a "separate-togetherness." However, like most other areas of couple life, it is imperative.

Kahlil Gibran wrote beautifully about this concept of "separate-togetherness" in his book *The Prophet*. Gibran's particular gift was in his choice of metaphors. The strings of the lute, he observed, though alone, "quiver with the same music." And while lovers should stand together, they should not be too near together, "for the pillars of the temple stand apart, and the oak tree and the cypress grow not in each other's shadow." The reason for all this is really quite clear. We are to love one another, "but make not a bond of love."

If you own a copy of *The Prophet*, read the passage I've referred to above; it is in the section on marriage. If you don't own a copy of the book, reflect on the metaphor of the strings on the lute, or the pillars of the temple. How do you embody this theme of separateness and togetherness in your own relationship? When you feel ready, do the exercise on the next page.

Exercise:
Separate Togetherness

Individually, each one of the couple draws a list of the activities, friends or other elements of their lives, noting whether the listings are separate or together. Once each list is drawn up, the couple will take time to share each other's assessment of their "separate-togetherness."

SEPARATE

1.

2.

3.

4.

5.

6.

7.

8.

9.

10.

TOGETHER

1.

2.

3.

4.

5.

6.

7.

8.

9.

10.

PRESCRIPTION: IT'S JUST A PHASE

In a couple relationship, there are four basic phases. Each phase has its own characteristics as well as time frame. This "phase" element in relationship explains why partners sometimes experience themselves differently or notice a shift in the way in which they are together, or apart. What are usually typical of each phase are the focus, the good and the bad, the style of communication and the overall character of the phase itself – in other words, what the phase feels like. On the next page, read through the brief explanation of each phase of relationship; an exercise will follow.

	VISIONARY	ADVERSARIAL	DORMANT	VITAL
FOCUS	us, and our future	you, your impact on me	me, interests that I find important	we, in the present
POSITIVE	a good start	potential for change	individual identity	combine forces
NEGATIVE	it won't last	win-lose,	disconnected	pair selfishness
STYLE OF COMMUNICATION	small talk, shop talk	fight-spite talk	small talk, shop talk	straight talk
CHARACTER	fantasy, playfulness, found "the" one	frustration, clear view, blame other	acceptance, functional emptiness	resilience, complemented relationship commitment

Note: For further reading on relationship phases I recommend *Connecting*, listed in the resources section at the end of this chapter.

Exercise

The exercise to accompany the "relationship phases" will be one that you will do over coffee. Choose a time when you are open to frank discussion with your partner. It is vital that each one of you take turns talking while the other listens and tries to understand what is being shared. In fact, this exercise is a sort of "can we talk?" activity. It will provide each of you with some degree of enlightenment as to which phase the other feels your relationship is in at present.

For discussion
"At present, I am experiencing our relationship in the... phase because..."

"Personally, my experience of this phase is…"

"If anything, I would like to see the following changes…"

When you have discussed the topics mentioned, you will have a clearer view of where you would like to go from here. Remember, there is help available from trained professionals whenever you find yourselves stuck somewhere or not knowing how to go about making the necessary changes.

Various couples report that their relationship has floated through the different stages, only to come back at times to one or the other. This can be a sign of growth and is perfectly healthy. We want always to maintain the uniqueness of each couple system and their experience of that system. For many couples, the parenting of their children affects their relationship phase; I encourage you to keep this in mind when you have discussions on this element of your coupleship.

PRESCRIPTION: PLAYING TOGETHER

One of the invigorating elements in an intimate partnership is play. Not only does it offer respite from stress, but it also effectively translates the validation that one partner can give to the other.

Some of us "adults" shy away from play because it brings forth our vulnerable self. We might have been programed into believing that the adult mode prohibits everything that is not serious and work related. Fortunately, the past few years have seen the emergence of adult play as an effective way to self-care.

The following are some examples of healthy adult play. I recommend them all to enhance the quality of your relationship. Feel free to create your own adult play; if you do so, you will be amazed at the creative energy you have as a legacy from your own inner child.

SWINGS: Take a walk in the park together and find the swings and the slides; enjoy each other's laughter as you play.

BATHTUB: Fill the tub with your favorite bubble bath; sit together in the tub, while you draw figures in the bubbles. It is a very soothing experience.

NICKNAMES: Call each other by a favorite nickname; be sure to check with your partner in case you might have chosen a nickname that he or she finds inappropriate.

EAT WITH YOUR FINGERS: Go out for your favorite finger foods. Personally, I adore nachos, loaded with "stuff." Eat from the same plate, with your fingers, and enjoy the freedom and the closeness of the experience.

GIFT FOR INNER CHILD: You may want to ask your partner if there was any toy or other type of gift that he or she wished for as a child but never received; your mission is then to surprise your lover with this specific gift if you can find it.

WATCH CARTOONS: Tune in to your favorite cartoons or rent a movie of them; make popcorn, have a pajama party or a picnic on the floor as you watch the entertainment.

SANDBOX: Find a sandbox in a playground; you might want to check that no other people are around, in case they find you a bit strange. When you have the privacy you want, dig in and have a contest as to who can build the best sand figure.

SWIMMING: There is something so uplifting about hearing the laughter of people playing in the water. Go swimming together, splash each other to your heart's content, show off your aquatic finesse to your partner. If you can find privacy, don't bother with bathing suits.

HALLOWEEN: Why should the kids get all the loot? Dress in a costume, grab your goodies bag and hit the pavement; a costume party or dance can fill the bill here as well.

PRESCRIPTION: CONFLICT RESOLUTION

"Marriage is the coming together of two unique and different individuals in order to share life with each other. Their differences are quite unavoidable. They have lived separate lives for perhaps 20 to 25 years, during which each has developed a set of individual tastes, preferences, habits, likes and dislikes, values and standards. It is totally unreasonable to suppose that two people, just because they are married to each other, should always want to do the same things in the same way at the same time."

(David and Vera Mace,
We Can Have Better Marriages If We Really Want Them)

CONFLICT is...
natural
a vital part of intimacy
inevitable in any relationship
a way to learn about me and you
handled in a positive way or in a negative way
a time for assertiveness, not aggressiveness
a time to remain calm
a source of vulnerability for some
sometimes brought on by resentment
an opportunity for strength and perseverance
a growth experience for a couple
often left unresolved
part of human relationships
often misunderstood or misinterpreted
mostly seen as anger which it is not
often treated with fear

perhaps a result of a bad past experience

a way of compromising

healthy in an intimate relationship

like the tension of violin strings

something to be mastered by effective technique

If a couple is seriously committed to working at their relationship, then each one will endeavor to learn how to resolve conflict. The following are suggested steps to follow, in chronological order, to effectively resolve a conflict.

Steps in Conflict Resolution

1. The issue
   - Be certain that both of you are clear on the issue that is the source of the conflict.
   - Zero in on the specific issue rather than draw all around it or bring in all sorts of other unfinished business.

2. Contract
   - Settle on a time frame to resolve conflict, do not exceed your time limit.
   - Choose a time and a place when you will do this.

3. Awareness
   - Here it is imperative that each of the partners tells how they experience the issue and the conflict; the other listens and attempts to understand what their partner is sharing.
   - There is no need to be in agreement, simply a great need to be heard and understood.

4. Wants
   - Take time to share with each other what you want as an outcome to this conflict.
   - Be respectful as you listen and try to understand your partner's point of view.

5. Options
   - It is important for each of us to feel that we have options and choices, no matter what the conflict is.

- List different options for a course of change or a course of action.
- An option could be status quo.
- This is not the time to choose one, but to simply brainstorm options.

6. Action
   - From the list of options you have drawn, you now agree on one choice of action.
   - Note that you can change your decision if at some point you realize that you have chosen an ineffective course of action.

7. Evaluate
   - Set a time and place when you will sit together to evaluate how your decision to resolve your conflict is coming along.
   - If it is working, applaud each other and celebrate.
   - If not, then simply go back to your list and try something else.

Note: For further reading and study on how to resolve conflict, I recommend *Talking and Listening Together* listed in the resources section at the end of this chapter.

Recommended Resources

1. Ables, Billie, S. *For Couples Only*
   Humanics New Age, Georgia, 1987
2. Beattie, Melody. *Codependent No More*
   Harper/Hazelden Books, San Francisco, 1987
3. Coché, Judith and Erich Coché. *Couples Groups*
   Brunner/Mazel Publishers, New York, 1990
4. Halpern, Howard. *How to Break Your Addiction to a Person*
   Bantam Books, New York, 1982
5. McKay, M., M. Davis, and P. Fanning. *Messages*
   New Harbinger Publications, 1983
6. Miller, Sherod, Daniel Wackman, Elam Nunally, and Phyllis Miller. *Connecting*
   Interpersonal Communications Programs Inc., CO, 1988
7. ———. *Talking and Listening Together,*
   Interpersonal Communications Programs Inc., CO, 1991
8. Sellner, Judith and James Sellner. *Between the Sexes*
   Self-Counsel Press Series, Toronto, 1986
9. Westheimer, Ruth. *Dr. Ruth's Guide for Married Lovers*
   Wings Books, New York, 1986
10. Young-Eisendrath, Polly. *Hags and Heroes*
    Inner City Books, Toronto, 1984

CHAPTER 11

DIVORCE/

BLENDED

FAMILIES

"I thought my gall bladder surgery had been a painful experience,
until I underwent divorce surgery; I thought that running a
marathon in my wheelchair was a challenge until I attempted to
create harmony within my blended family."
– Louise Giroux

Divorce is a surgical procedure. Blended families face intense challenges. Somehow, the two often accompany one another. Since the divorce process goes on for many years, if not for an entire lifetime, when people incorporate a blended family system into their lives, they experience compounded stress. From my own experience and from that of many of my clients, from whom I have had the privilege to learn, I can attest to the necessity for a couple to prepare, and to go slowly and cautiously. They need to seek help and support not only during a divorce but also during the first years in the life of a new blended family. This chapter will offer a few suggestions and activities designed to make the experience of divorce and of the blended family more livable.

CASE STUDY

Sandra appears apprehensive and nervous for her first session with the therapist. For almost an hour, she pours out the story of what her life has been like since her divorce, almost two years ago. It contains a mixture of grieving her first marriage, letting go of her first husband, falling in love with a new husband and the instant family that both this new partner and she have been gifted with. It's all too much for her to handle.

The therapist strives to get her to focus on one issue at a time, starting with the divorce. How has her grieving been going? Sandra reports that, at first, any verbal contact with Tim was a shouting match. Because she had custody of their children, Tim feared she would alienate them from him. Once he realized that she wasn't going to do this, they seem to have gradually reached a level of new comfort. To the therapist's delight, Sandra talks about how she and the children's father can celebrate birthdays together now; there seems to be an effort on everyone's part to enjoy each other whenever possible and to focus on the good memories.

It appears that her new blended family is the most stressful issue for Sandra at present. John and she have a seemingly healthy relationship, both of them enjoying this marriage to each other. Because both have experienced marriage warfare in their first marriages, they are prepared, willing and committed to build a solid relationship with each other. The problem is with the children. Sandra brings a son and a daughter into the blended family; John brings two sons. Instantly, all members, parents and children, are parachuted into this new system for which they were not prepared.

The four children range in ages from 27 to 12. Richard is the eldest, now 27, married and living in another city; his brother Andrew is 22, presently enrolled in a third year at university; these two brothers are John's sons from his first marriage. Paul is 16, in grade eleven and living with Sandra and John, as is Melody, the youngest member of the new family, a 12-year-old.

Through an outpouring of tears, Sandra talks about how dreadful it has been trying to find some harmony in this new blended family. Richard is unaccepting of his father's new wife; he is almost totally estranged from his father. For Andrew, it is a case of rebellion; he doesn't want much to do with his father or his new wife or her children; his dad's lectures have left him disenchanted with the new blended family. Andrew knows how to solve everyone's relational problems. Paul is an obnoxious teenager; when John tries to discipline him, Paul becomes unbearable. There are times when Sandra fears that the two will turn to physical violence. Amazingly enough, Paul and John get along quite well when they spend time alone. What keeps Sandra from giving up on this new blended family is the rapport that John has with Melody. Still young enough to be influenced and easy enough to handle, Melody accepts John readily and assesses that her mother has never been happier.

At the end of this first session, the therapist takes over and tries to encourage Sandra and to offer some explanations as to what is transpiring as well as some course of treatment for the situation. Jealousy, anger, emotional outbursts, isolation and rebellion are all part of the first stages of a new blended family coming together. A reasonable amount of pressure must be exerted by all members on each other to invite them to join together without, at the same time, making unreasonable demands on them. Each child is reacting individually to this new parenting and simultaneously grieving the loss of the former nuclear family. They may be experiencing a certain level of anxiety regarding their loyalties to their biological parents. One thing is certain; things can improve and should improve if the members are willing to work at it. Sandra is greatly relieved when she books another appointment for herself with the therapist. Following this, the therapist will spend some session-time with each member of the family and then proceed to do some family system therapy for the entire family.

EXERCISE IN SONG

The selected song for this chapter is *You've Lost That Loving Feeling,* by The Righteous Brothers.

In all divorce situations there are losses and there are gains. Fill the balance sheet that follows to get a clearer sense of the reasons for your marriage breakdown.

_____and_____

BALANCE SHEET FOR MARRIAGE ENDING _____

ASSETS (Gains)

_____ +

_____ +

_____ +

_____ +

_____ +

_____ +

TOTAL ASSETS _____ +

LIABILITIES (Losses)

_____ –

_____ –

_____ –

_____ –

_____ –

_____ –

TOTAL LIABILITIES _____ –

BALANCE OF LIABILITIES AND ASSETS _____

Exercise in Film

The film selection for this chapter is *Kramer vs. Kramer*. Although the film is now several years old, in my opinion it portrays very effectively the turmoil associated with marriage breakdown. In this particular case, the turmoil mushrooms into a child custody conflict. As you view the film, think of the experience lived by the characters.

THE KRAMER SYSTEM

Ted   Joanna

    Billy

1. In the Kramer family system, how do each of the three members experience the separation/divorce and battle?

2. Imagine you are Joanna and build a case for yourself and your decision.

3. Imagine you are Ted and build a defense for yourself.

4. If Billy could express himself as an adult, what might he want and need to communicate to his parents?

5. Margaret, Joanna's friend, is somehow involved in the process; how do you see her involvement?

6. After seeing this film, what are some of the learnings that you have collected for yourself?

Exercise:
Sit Down and Write a Letter

Write a good-bye letter to your former partner. The intent is to focus on positive memories and gratitude for whatever was good in your relationship. I recommend that you express this intent to him or to her so as to avoid the possibility of false expectations. This is an exercise for your grieving growth, therefore the outcome is irrelevant. What matters most is for you to do it.

PRESCRIPTION: DEAR LOU...

THURSDAY, SEPTEMBER 1, 199_

THE GAZETTE

Dear Lou...

My parents have been divorced for well over five years now. At the beginning we all had to get over it, if you know what I mean. At that time, I felt pretty good about it because neither one of them ever questioned me about what the other was up to. I am living in residence and thankful that I never had to live with either one of them since their divorce.

About one year ago, my mother got a boyfriend who has since become a live-in; that's no big deal in itself. He's fine with me and she seems happier. It's my father who drives me crazy. Each time I talk with him, he interrogates me on what my mother is up to. He even asks dumb questions about their sex life, as if I care or want to discuss that with him.

I have spoken to my mother about him and she cannot seem to help me; she says she has to keep out of it, I mean the relationship between my dad and me. When the phone rings late at night, I just know it's my father pumping me for information. I encouraged him to get on with his life and even tried to set him up with a woman. He refused... I really have my own life to live, I'm in third year economics and I don't need my parents tearing me apart like this. Can you help me?

Signed,
Caught-in-the-middle

EXERCISE

Answer for Dear Lou with all the expertise Lou has on these types of situations.

Dear Caught-in-the-middle,

Signed,

Lou

EXERCISE: CINDERELLA

Mothers have often been given a bad name; especially "step"mothers. Some of this has been the consequence of myths as well as stereotyping. The following exercise might clear up some of the issues around your parenting if you have children in your blended family.

Read or watch *Cinderella* with your children; make it a family type of activity and as enjoyable as possible. By the way, I believe that fairy tales are for audiences of every age. After you have read it or watched it, discuss the stereotype of the wicked stepmother as well as how it applies to your family system or not. It is important that the children, no matter how young, be heard.

EXERCISE: OUR FAMILY ALBUM

Because a blended family must make its identity from its own essence and character, it is imperative to accomplish certain tasks and also to enjoy certain activities as a whole system. The new family must integrate and blend if it is to function cohesively. It is, however, counterproductive to use rigidity or pressure. I recommend a smooth approach creating an *invitation* to belong. Keep in mind that teenagers can cause havoc, simply because they are teenagers. Their sense of loyalties may be confused and their need to individuate very strong.

EXERCISE

Make a family album. Invite all the members of your new blended family to participate. I recommend that you call "Johnny" *our* son, rather than your husband's son, and so on.

Prescription:
Stages in Blended Family

THE BEGINNING

Where are we...?

This stage lasts anywhere from one to four years depending on circumstances and willingness of those involved to make it work.

Here's the picture...
- Contact between the children and their non-custodial parent is conflicted.
- The ex-spouses are in their "settling" phase.
- The new parent comes to the rescue.
- Hope is restored that they will be a new family.
- Children ignore the new parent or make their lives a living hell, hoping that he or she will go away.
- Members live with confusion, shame and inadequacy.
- Loyalty pulls are rampant.

Recipe for survival...
- Allow as long as it takes for all members to effectively grieve their losses, remembering that usually a child, no matter what their age, wants their biological parents together.
- Encourage openness of all members as to how they are experiencing this new family.
- Accept that a new blended family does not magically live in harmony (sorry, there is no real *Brady Bunch*).
- Be prepared to wait it out.

THE MIDDLE

Where are we...?

This is the stage for boundary setting, that is, the establishing of effective limits – lasts anywhere from two to three years.

Here's the picture...
- More and more the children set new healthy boundaries with their non-custodial parent.
- Ex-spouses by this time have sorted out many of their differences.

- Members mobilize around the new blended family's needs.
- Persons begin to work as a team.
- Boundaries are set: the couple negotiate their parenting.
- The ex-spouse respects the new system and stops the sabotaging.
- The new blended family begins to take shape, with its own specific character.

Recipe for survival...
- Provide as much accessibility to the non-custodial parent as is healthy.
- Validate your ex-spouse for their respect of your new system.
- Hold family meetings often to invite open sharing.
- Get together as parents in a blended system to evaluate and thank each other for help.
- Schedule outings, phone calls, photos – any activity that will maintain the cohesion of your family system.

THE END
Where are we...?
Finally we have arrived. The blended family reaches a healthy degree of cohesiveness. This stage usually lasts from one to two years and reaches far beyond.

Here's the picture...
- A mature new family system emerges.
- There is a fluctuation of ups and downs, as there is in any family system.
- Children experience two family households; often they can go back and forth without major upheaval and they have adapted to the different rules and atmosphere of each home.
- Co-parenting is a consultation between the ex-spouse and the parents in the blended family; there is a harmony where the children are concerned.
- An intimacy begins to develop between the children and the new parent.
- All roles become much clearer.

Recipe for survival...
- Welcome your new family system's life.
- Be realistic in your expectations.
- Express pride in the children's growth during the ordeal of adjustment.

- Thank the ex-spouse for their integration of the new blended family into their life.
- Co-parent with the ex-spouses since you never divorced the children.
- Do not fear the new intimacy: new systems are often frightening since people are afraid of a repeat performance of the first family.
- Remember to party together, eat together, sing and dance, as well as cry together.
- Remain open with each other.

Note: Just as all stages in any experience are characterized by individual variants, it is such for the stages that make up the building of a new blended family system. In some cases, very little time and energy may be expended while with others, it may take forever to reach a new growth or it may simply never happen.

EXERCISE

Think and chart how your grief stages developed in the blended family system. In the left column are the members of your system; adapt to your own constellation. The three other columns refer to the three steps in the different stages: "Where are we...? Here's the picture... and Recipe for survival..."

	WHERE I AM	PICTURE	SURVIVAL
MEMBER 1			
MEMBER 2			
MEMBER 3			
MEMBER 4			
MEMBER 5			
MEMBER 6			
MEMBER 7			

RECOMMENDED RESOURCES

1. Ahrons, Constance and Roy H. Rodgers. *Divorced Families*
   W.W. Norton & Company, New York, 1987
2. Beavers, W. Robert and Robert B. Hampson. *Successful Families*
   W.W. Norton & Company, New York, 1990
3. Felder, Leonard. *A Fresh Start*
   Penguin Books, New York, 1987
4. Kahn, Sandra S. *Ex-Wife Syndrome*
   Random House, New York, 1990
5. Kalter, Neil. *Growing Up with Divorce*
   Fawcett Columbine, New York, 1990
6. Krantzler, Mel. *Creative Divorce*
   A Signet Book, New American Library, 1973
7. Morrison, Kati. *Stepmothers, Exploring the Myth*
   Canadian Council on Social Development, Ottawa, 1986
8. Peck, Scott. *The Road Less Travelled*
   Simon and Schuster, New York, 1978
9. Wallerstein, Judith & Sandra Blakeslee. *Second Chances*
   Ticknor and Fields, New York, 1989

CHAPTER 12

RECYCLING

THE CIRCLE

"Within the profound experience of the self-recycled, is born the infinity of the circle of life."

– Louise Giroux

The final chapter of this workbook deals with ways in which we can enhance our quality of life constantly. In the circle of life, we are shaped and blended to assert our uniqueness as well as our sameness with our fellow humans. I believe that one of the reasons why people become "life-less" is that they forget or simply do not know how to "recycle" themselves. It brings to mind the taste of a little horseradish on gefilte fish...mmm...just enough spice brings life to the food.

Do you have a green thumb? Most people do; this chapter will talk about plants and their special life energy. What about a dog? Even though dogs are kids in fur coats, needing a lot of care, they are a magic animal for us. How many true friends can you count on in your life? Have you ever taken the time to light candles and watch them? This chapter will invite you to drive a Rolls-Royce. (Now I'm *sure* I have your attention.) Is there a soul mate for you in your life or are you settling for less because you think you're not worth more? Do you have a G – d concept that works for you?

These are some of the areas that will be dealt with.

CASE STUDY

The case study for this final chapter of the workbook is my own story. Please refer to my autobiography, *RECYCLED: A Story of Hope*, which may be obtained through the publisher:
FENIX RYZING ASSOCIATES
Box 172 Station. Q, Toronto, Ontario Canada M4T 2M1

Because this chapter wraps everything together in the "Recycling the Circle of Life" theme, I thought that my case study would be appropriate.

At a time in my adult life, when everything "should" have been stable, my world fell apart; I entered this painstaking process of recycling, a totally broken person. In my case, a chronic illness precipitated the recycling, which had begun in a subdued way, a few years prior in different aspects of my life.

Anything from a new hobby, to a child leaving home, to mid-life crisis, may act as a catalyst in the process of recycling our life. Although the precipitating incident may vary, in all cases a bankruptcy of our life, as we know it, must occur. This state of crisis manifests itself financially, emotionally, spiritually or physically and is, in effect, the energizing force for the recycling process.

For the next few years following the "crash," I dug up the skeletons. My mother, who died when I was 13, had a great deal to do with my identity as a woman, so I searched to know her better. I had been daddy's girl; my relationship with my father fell nothing short of enmeshed and pathological; it needed to be treated since all my relationships with males were under its influence.

My father had the same chronic illness that I was now diagnosed with; how would I walk my own path with my illness and not follow my father's? I was the mother of a seven-year-old. The way I had been parented had everything to do with the type of parent I had become; how effective was I? My marriage was broken yet I remained for fear of taking the giant step toward standing on my own. Because of my illness, my career, as I knew it, ended abruptly; at age 36, I imprisoned myself in my home.

Any faith or spiritual life perished under the burden of depression and rage. Either I recycled myself, or I died. I chose to live.

Extracted from who I was, made new and improved through self-awareness, self-reclaiming and self-creation: "I am recycled."

EXERCISE IN SONG

The song for this exercise is Elton John's *Circle of Life* from the film *The Lion King*.

Write a piece on the following topic: "This is my place in the Circle of Life." Attempt to express your inner thoughts and feelings.

THIS IS MY PLACE IN THE CIRCLE OF LIFE

THIS IS MY PLACE IN THE CIRCLE OF LIFE

Exercise in Film

The Lion King was the blockbuster film of the summer of '94 and one of the most moving films I have ever viewed. After seeing it three times, I would see it again in a wink. Not only is it an artful production in aesthetic cartooning but it also speaks of the profound truth about recycling our lives and participating in the circle of life. Enjoy viewing this film and do the exercise that follows.

This exercise deals with the character sketches presented in the movie. Each of the animals represents a type of person, with their own life experience. For example, Rafiki, the monkey, is an animated representation of the wise counselor or the clergy person who sees beyond the obvious. Fill in the following "character sketches" as well as "what I learned" for the movie's characters. For example, from Rafiki, you might have learned the value of a spiritual mentor in your life.

Who	Type of person animated	What I learned
MUFASA		
RAFIKI		
SCAR		
QUEEN SARABI		
SIMBA		
ZAZU		

Who	Type of person animated	What I learned
PUMBAA		
TIMON		
NALA		
BANZAI, SHENZI and ED		

PRESCRIPTION: ADOPT PLANTS

The more you surround yourself with life energy, the more you will find your individual place in the circle of life as well as a profound peace within your soul. Plants are life energy. Not only do they adorn with visual beauty, but they represent growth: a cycle of growth that we can see before our very eyes. Like us, plants are repeatedly renewed with the sun's energy and with water. A few dollars is all that is needed to adopt plants for your home or office.

Instructions

1. Adopt a plant.
2. Name her and use her name to speak to her and to care for her.
3. Introduce her to family and friends.
4. Familiarize yourself with her specific needs in terms of light and water.
5. Display her where she can be a part of your visual surroundings: show her off !!!
6. As she grows and emanates ENERGY, thank her for sharing her beauty and aliveness with you.
7. Keep her hair (branches and leaves or flowers) healthy and in a style

suitable to her personality; prepare her before her haircuts so as not to shock her.

8. If she blesses you with babies, adopt them also or offer them to others.
9. RECYCLE LIFE ENERGY.

PRESCRIPTION:
FALL IN LOVE WITH A DOG

"...to form a friendship that at its profoundest moments has need of neither words nor outward signs..."

      – Ulrich Klever, *The Complete Book of Dog Care*

What you put into it
- money to purchase or adopt a dog, or two, or three...
- time spent training the dog
- frustration at picking up the doggy doo
- annoyance at the barking
- money for dog food and other supplies
- expenses for the vet
- a baby sitter once in a while

What you get out of it
- a true friend
- a family network
- great recreation
- exercise for your back
- a guard for your home
- an eater of leftovers
- a great caretaker when you are ill
- the most charming face
- laughter at dog tricks
- a foot warmer
- a live, huggable, plush toy
- unconditional love
- unconditional affection
- unconditional acceptance

EXERCISE: YOU'VE GOT A FRIEND

To do this exercise on true friendship, I suggest you listen to the song *You've Got a Friend*, recorded by Carole King and by James Taylor. After you do so, answer the following questions.

1. According to experts, a person is considered lucky if they have three true friendships. How many do you have?

2. How do you maintain your friendships?

3. Do your friendships last?

4. Are your friendships strong enough to withstand healthy conflict?

5. If you were dying and needed to leave your child in the care of a friend, whom would you choose and why?

6. If you were stuck on an island, with which one of your friends would you prefer to be?

7. Do your friends consider you their true friend?

8. If you are unsatisfied with your true friendship, what could you do about it?

Prescription: Light Candles

Candles and flame are life energy just as plants are. What fascinates me is the warmth and the strength of the flame. I use it for anchoring, that is, for focusing myself, a technique popularly used by therapists and religious contemplatives. Entering into its breathing, I visualize it entering into me and anchoring into me as I feel a sense of warmth, a sense of light. Mostly, it is the aliveness of the flame that intrigues me.

When you watch a candle, it dances, it moves and just when you think that it is about to die, it rises from its ashes like a phoenix. Candles and flame help people to celebrate. If you give a candle to someone, when you light that other person's flame with your own flame, you lose nothing, in fact you form a network.

Materials
candles
matches
willing participant
a relaxing few moments

Instructions
light your favorite candle (scented candles reach the senses better)
turn off the electric lights
relax your body by taking deep breaths
watch the flame
think calming, loving thoughts
when you finish you will feel totally refreshed
don't burn your candle at both ends

PRESCRIPTION:
DRIVE A ROLLS-ROYCE

There is something to be said for living out one's fantasies. If you can fulfill one of your dreams you will be amazed at the therapeutic value of the experience. Once again, keep in mind that expectations are to be kept to an appropriate level. Also, you will want to be logical and not spend money that you cannot afford to spend. Many fantasies are livable, if you make a few concessions and adaptations. Here is an interesting dream come true for Sarah.

NAME: Sarah

DESCRIPTION: Caucasian, 43 years old, brown eyes, brown hair

WEIGHT: acceptable and appropriate

CAREER: social worker and domestic engineer

FAMILY CONSTELLATION: blended family with three children

$ STATUS: average middle-class

TEMPERAMENT: intense, creative and somewhat depressive

DIAGNOSIS: Feeling of "blue" intensified by the fact that Sarah comes to the realization that she will never be able to afford the Rolls-Royce she has always dreamt of driving.

TREATMENT: rent a Rolls-Royce and drive it around

PROGNOSIS: Excellent. Sarah will undoubtedly get a kick and fulfill a fantasy. She will be able to say, "When I drove my Rolls..."

MY PROFILE AND FANTASY

NAME:

DESCRIPTION:

WEIGHT:

CAREER:

FAMILY CONSTELLATION:

$ STATUS:

TEMPERAMENT:

DIAGNOSIS:

TREATMENT:

PROGNOSIS:

PRESCRIPTION: WHERE ART THOU, MY SOUL MATE...?

Definitions (from Webster's New Collegiate Dictioinary, 1976)

MATE: (1) associate companion (2) an assistant to a more skilled workman (3) one of a pair as either member of a married couple (4) equal match (5) to join together as mates (6) one of two persons temperamentally suited to each other

SOUL: (1) the immaterial essence, animating principle, or actuating cause of an individual life (2) the spiritual principle embodied in human beings, all rational and spiritual beings, or the universe (3) a person's total self (4) a moving spirit

I would hope that you are gifted with a soul mate in your life. If you are, then celebrate them; if you have a soul mate "in the making," validate him or her and enjoy each other; if you are alone, set your sights on the fact that you are worthy of a soul mate and don't settle for anything less. Realize that you may be better off alone than in relationship with someone who isn't compatible.

EXERCISE

Compose an ad for the personal classifieds in which you capture the essence of what a soul mate means to you.

THE GAZETTE

Companions

_____

_____

_____

_____

_____

_____

_____

_____

_____

_____

_____

_____

_____

_____

_____

_____

_____

_____

_____

_____

_____

_____

Prescription:
Meditate with Quotations

One of the ways in which you can energize your life is by a simple meditative technique. You can use famous or not-so-famous quotations that speak in some way to you. I suggest you simply take a few moments every morning, since it is the "stage-setting" time for your day; read a quotation and take time to reflect on its message for you at this particular moment. You can make use of the popular meditation books or simply thumb through your favorite book. Remain in a thinking and feeling mode while you read the quotation over a few times. The awareness and the calm that is rejuvenated from this time for meditation will be a great asset to you in your everyday life.

Some quotations

"I learned how to survive, but not how to live." – Gilly A.

"I haven't won yet but I haven't lost." – Dennis C.

"Life is not a problem to be solved, but a reality to be experienced."
– S. Kierkegaard

"Others will mostly treat you the way you treat yourself." – M. Moussa

"Because I have been athirst, I will dig a well that others may drink."
– Arabian Proverb

"Resolve to be thyself; and know that who finds himself, loses his misery."
– Matthew Arnold

"At 70, my dad is just like he was at 35 – only more so. It's frightening that the same thing could happen to me." – Jerry Z.

"You love me so much, you want to put me in your pocket. And I should die there smothered." – D. H. Lawrence

"When I grow up, I want to be a child." – Dick H.

"I am not responsible for my feelings – only for what I do with them."
– Dr. Ceophus Martin

PRESCRIPTION:
THE CIRCLE OF LIFE

The Circle
dedicated to Adam-Paul

He gurgles...and in strange sounds his mother hears a love song, an ode to mother and child. She sits by his crib, watching him as he sleeps. "My angel," she whispers, "You are so beautiful my precious one." In the perfectly contented face of the infant, the world is transformed for her.

He reaches on tiptoe to switch on the stereo. The mother jumps at the shriek of the "ten" volume control only to applaud her son's determination in finally reaching the on and off switch. In a swaying embrace, they dance together; the more mommy spins her toddler around, the more he laughs. As they spin around the room, her world is full... abundant with her knowledge that her son is inquisitive and resourceful.

The autumn hue decorates the woody path. As the mother takes her toddler's hand, he breaks free of her. In the moment that pauses the frame of the action in her whole world, the son begins to walk. After each stagger and fall, he re-takes his walking and laughs out loud at his new-found freedom. The mother knows that her son has taken his giant step in becoming his own person.

She watches from her parked car as her little boy makes his way into the school. On his back, he proudly carries a "Star Wars" school bag. "He is so small, so young," his mother whispers to herself. She wipes a tear, one that connects her mother's heart to the reality that she will have her son less and less with her.

The pride in her heart overwhelms her as she sits among the audience. "I will now play *Barcarole*," he speaks in a thick French accent. In spite of the less than perfect interpretation of the musical number, the audience applauds and he takes a bow. The accordion is half his size. She cannot focus her camera because of the tears in her eyes; her heart hears the music of her grandfather, of her mother, of herself playing the piano and of this little son making his debut in music.

If the mosquitoes were not so thick, this night would be perfect. She doesn't mind the uncomfortable seat in the bleachers, because her son has pitched an excellent game. The other parents all know him and cheer him on; she has been warned by him not to make such a fuss when he lands a great one. Tomorrow, his team leaves for a tournament; they will travel four hundred miles. She will worry and so her son promises to call her every night while he is gone.

This must be the hundredth balloon she is blowing up as she glances at the gorgeous cake; it reads, "Happy teen-hood my son." Soon his friends will arrive; that is when she will disappear behind the scenes since he has asked for the "no-mom" thing while he parties with them. She wonders how they can understand anything at all from the blaring music while they all seem to enjoy it tremendously.

How could this happen! The pain in her side is excruciating but not as much as the pain of knowing that she cannot deliver the speech she has prepared for the event. When her son comes up with the idea that he will deliver the speech for her, she sobs. He doesn't understand why until she asks, "You will do this for me?" It is a mixture of pride, of gratitude, of anxiousness and of deep love that lifts her pain from her as he leaves her hospital room. Her son is becoming an integrated person.

She watches from the window as he gets into the car; he has been a licensed driver for all of eight hours. In harmony with the sound of the ignition, her heart beats with a new pride as well as a new fear. Her mind races to catch up with the actuality of her son's independence. It seems it was just yesterday when she carried him out of the car and secured him in his car seat; today, he is driving away. Her motherly love overwhelms her...she is breathless.

From her seat in the auditorium, she catches sight of her son who, in a few moments, will be a university graduate. The stage is full to the brim yet among the few hundred mortarboards, she only has eyes for one red-haired man. As he advances to receive his diploma his mother's eyes and his eyes meet and in her motherly loving voice, the son hears, "I am so very proud of you my son."

There is an air of shyness as he introduces his new girlfriend to his mother. One immediately determines that this girl is bright and well grounded. It is mostly small talk around the table as the two women get acquainted; when the younger one leaves the table, the son whispers lovingly to his mom, "There goes the girl I am going to marry." The mother smiles at her son who has become a young lover.

The telephone ring wakes her with the sound of her son's voice, "He looks just like me, Mom." She feels older for a moment; her motherly love transforms into grandmotherly love and she cries. Now there is another baby to love, to watch, to enjoy. Quickly she hops out of bed, only to race to the side of her son and his newborn baby. He gurgles....

EXERCISE

Write a brief story of your own and title it "The Circle." Share the story with your children, if you have any, since they are usually thrilled at hearing or reading about how they are part of our life cycle, life circle, life recycling.

The Circle

The Circle

PRESCRIPTION:
CONNECT WITH A G — D

Assuming that you have incorporated a G – d-like concept in your life, one technique whereby you can get relief from worry and overfunctioning, is what I call a G – d box.

Materials

a small decorative box
a piece of paper and a pencil
an issue that you need relief from

Instructions

1. Design your own G – d box. Choose whatever expresses your uniqueness.
2. Label your G – d box with something like this, "_____'s G – d box; I can let go of whatever is in here because it is being taken care of."
3. When you feel a need to let go of an issue, write it briefly on a piece of paper; fold it and retire it to your G – d box. It has left you for now and it is being dealt with. Putting in a number of issues on separate pieces of paper is also recommended. There is no limit to how much your G – d box can hold safely.

If you have difficulty connecting with G – d because you've lost G – d's address and phone number, and you don't have access to a fax, think about the following quotation in which the consonants YHWH stand for the Hebrew name of G – d:

> ...he discovered YHWH, not in awesome manifestations of nature, like a devastating wind, an earthquake, a sudden fire, but in the still small voice that is the unyielding strength of every man of vision. Not the external world of nature but the inner, intangible, unseen groping of man toward spiritual and moral awareness... that is where YHWH is to be found.
>
> – Chaim Potok, *Wanderings*

PRESCRIPTION: LIVING WHOLE

You have probably heard someone say, "Something is missing in my life." This statement expresses the status of "un-wholeness," that is, the person is not fulfilled in the six parts of wholeness. Clinebell* speaks of the six dimensions of wholeness that we need to develop in order to experience life fully. This is an adaptation of these six dimensions.

The Six Dimensions of Wholeness

1. Psychological: Enlivening one's mind. Involves developing our rich, partially-used, personality resources for thinking, feeling, experiencing, envisioning and creating.

2. Physical: Revitalizing one's body. This means learning to experience and enjoy one's body more fully, and to use it more effectively and lovingly.

3. Interpersonal: Renewing and enriching one's intimate relationships. This involves helping people to repair, renew and enrich their network of caring relationships.

4. Environmental: Deepening one's relationship with nature and the biosphere. This involves increasing our ecological awareness by communing with and caring about, as well as nurturing interaction with our great mother – Mother Nature.

5. Institutional: Growth in relation to the significant institutions in one's life. To aim at freeing, motivating and empowering ourselves to work with others to make our institutions places where wholeness will be better nurtured in everyone.

6. Spiritual: Deepening and vitalizing one's relationship with G – d. This dimension intersects and unifies the other five providing an open, trustful, nourishing, joy-full relationship with the loving Spirit who is the source of all life, all healing, all growth.

*adapted from *Basic Types of Pastoral Care and Counselling*

EXERCISE: MY WHOLENESS

This is a writing exercise. Complete the following sentences to the best of your ability.

In the psychological dimension, I have...

and I need to...

In the physical dimension, I have...

and I need to...

In the interpersonal dimension, I have...

and I need to...

In the environmental dimension I have...

and I need to...

In the institutional dimension I have...

and I need to...

In the spiritual dimension I have...

and I need to...

Recommended Resources

1. Bach, Richard. *Jonathan Livingston Seagull*
   Avon Books, New York, 1973
2. Bristol, Claude. *The Magic of Believing*
   Pocket Books, New York, 1948
3. Casey, Karen. *The Love Book*
   Hazelden Foundation, U.S.A., 1985
4. Clinebell, Howard. *Basic Types of Pastoral Care and Counselling*
   Welch Publishing Company, Burlington, Ontario, 1989
5. Cordes, Liane. *The Reflecting Pond*
   Hazelden Meditation Series, U.S.A., 1981
6. Fynn. *Mister God, This Is Anna*
   Ballantine Books, New York, 1974
7. Goldhor Lerner, Harriet. *The Dance of Intimacy*
   Harper and Row Publishers, New York, 1989
8. Greenwald, Jerry. *Be the Person You Were Meant to Be*
   Dell Publishing, New York, 1973
9. Jampolsky, Gerald. *Teach Only Love*
   Bantam Books, Toronto, 1983
10. Keating, Kathleen. *The Hug Therapy Book*
    Comp Care Publications, Minnesota, 1983
11. Kushner, Harold. *To Life!*
    Little Brown and Company, Toronto, 1993
12. Lembo, John. *Help Yourself*
    Argus Communications, Illinois, 1974
13. LeShan, Lawrence. *How to Meditate*
    Bantam Books, New York, 1974
14. Levin, Pamela. *Becoming the Way We Are*
    Health Communications Inc., Florida, 1974
15. ———. *Cycles of Power*
    Health Communications, Florida, 1988
16. Lindquist, Marie. *Holding Back*
    Hazelden Foundation, 1987
17. O'Connor, Dagmar. *How to Put the Love Back into Making Love*
    Doubleday Publishers, 1989
18. Powell, John. *The Secret of Staying in Love*
    Tabor Publishing, CA, 1974
19. ———. *Why Am I Afraid to Tell You Who I Am?*
    Argus Communications, Texas, 1969
20. Robben, John. *Coming to my Senses*
    Ballantine Books, 1973
21. Shaw, Leonard. *Love and Forgiveness*
    Leonard Shaw Publishers, 1989
22. Tweski, Abraham. *Waking Up Just in Time*
    Topper Books, New York, 1990

A THOUGHT FOR

THE JOURNEY

I hope you have learned much, enjoyed much, and healed much as you have worked through the pages of this book. The journey of healing is, of course, an ongoing one. As you continue to work at your own healing, I would remind you of this final bit of wisdom:

"Nothing is impossible...it's just that I haven't done it yet."